HEARING LOSS

Questions
you
have
. . . Answers
you
need

Other Books From The People's Medical Society

Take This Book to the Hospital With You

How to Evaluate and Select a Nursing Home

Medicine on Trial

Medicare Made Easy

Your Medical Rights

Getting the Most for Your Medical Dollar

Take This Book to the Gynecologist With You

Take This Book to the Obstetrician With You

Blood Pressure: Questions You Have . . . Answers You Need

Your Heart: Questions You Have . . . Answers You Need

The Consumer's Guide to Medical Lingo

150 Ways to Be a Savvy Medical Consumer

Take This Book to the Pediatrician With You

100 Ways to Live to 100

Dial 800 for Health

Your Complete Medical Record

Arthritis: Questions You Have . . . Answers You Need

Diabetes: Questions You Have . . . Answers You Need

Prostate: Questions You Have . . . Answers You Need

Vitamins and Minerals: Questions You Have . . . Answers You Need

Good Operations—Bad Operations

The Complete Book of Relaxation Techniques

Test Yourself for Maximum Health

Misdiagnosis: Woman As a Disease

Yoga Made Easy

Asthma: Questions You Have . . . Answers You Need

HEARING LOSS

Questions
you
have
...Answers
you
need

By Jennifer Hay

≡People's Medical Society®
Allentown, Pennsylvania

The People's Medical Society is a nonprofit consumer health organization dedicated to the principles of better, more responsive and less expensive medical care. Organized in 1983, the People's Medical Society puts previously unavailable medical information into the hands of consumers so that they can make informed decisions about their own health care.

Membership in the People's Medical Society is $20 a year and includes a subscription to the *People's Medical Society Newsletter.* For information, write to the People's Medical Society, 462 Walnut Street, Allentown, PA 18102, or call 610 770-1670.

This and other People's Medical Society publications are available for quantity purchase at discount. Contact the People's Medical Society for details.

Library of Congress Cataloging-in-Publication Data
Hay, Jennifer, 1964–
    Hearing loss : questions you have—answers you need /
by Jennifer Hay.
        p. cm.
    Includes bibliographical references and index.
    ISBN 1-882606-15-9
    1. Deafness—Miscellanea.   2. Deafness—Popular works.
I. Title.
RF291.35.H39   1994
617.8—dc20
                                        94-30069
                                            CIP

    3 4 5 6 7 8 9 0
First printing, August 1994

CONTENTS

INTRODUCTION

When I was a small child, I remember seeing people my grandparents' age with silver, rectangular boxes hanging around their necks. Leading from the box was a wire that led to a plug-like device that shoved into the ear. This was the "modern" hearing aid.

That was back in the 1950s. And both the technology and science relating to hearing loss were fairly primitive. Since those days, both science and technology have made quantum leaps. We know so much more about the causes and types of hearing loss. We understand better how sound and hearing work. Modern engineering, space-age materials, miniaturization and computerization have turned the hearing aid, which began as a simple ear trumpet, into a sophisticated, adaptive device that has reopened the world for many millions of people.

Hearing loss is as common as a roomful of people. It affects all age groups. Some people are born with it. Others suffer from it as a result of an injury or disease. Still others observe its onset as they age. The bad news about hearing loss is that it is occurring more frequently as people live longer, noise levels increase and other environmental factors take hold. The good news is that there are some solid strategies that can help prevent it from occurring and many excellent devices, interventions and personal environmental approaches that can lessen its impact. There are even some relatively new surgical procedures that may help restore hearing.

Hearing Loss: Questions You Have . . . Answers You Need covers all the important facts you need to know about hearing loss itself and the devices and treatments available. In an easy-to-read, question-and-answer format, the book guides you through the most commonly asked questions.

Hearing loss has become an industry in America. Hearing aids are often sold in stores by persons who have no training whatsoever. Most states do little to regulate the sale of hearing devices, those qualified to sell them or how safe and effective the product itself may be. Because of this, many consumers are often misdiagnosed or are sold products that can do little or nothing to restore hearing, or they even may end up totally confused and many dollars poorer.

That is why *Hearing Loss: Questions You Have . . . Answers You Need* is an essential part of your hearing health care.

As the nation's largest consumer health advocacy organization, the nonprofit People's Medical Society is dedicated to getting helpful and healthful information to the consumer. It is our philosophy that an informed consumer is an empowered one—a person capable of making the best health-care decisions in partnership with her health-care provider.

Thus, the more you know about hearing loss and the products and services available to ease its burden, the more likely you will be to find useful and significant help.

Charles B. Inlander
President, People's Medical Society

HEARING LOSS

**Questions
you
have
... Answers
you
need**

Terms printed in boldface can be found in the glossary, beginning on page 157. Only the first mention of the word in the text will be boldfaced.

We have tried to use male and female pronouns in an egalitarian manner throughout the book. Any imbalance in usage has been in the interest of readability.

1 SOUND INFORMATION

Q: What is hearing?

A: Hearing, one of the five senses, is the ability to perceive and interpret sound.

Q: So hearing loss is . . . ?

A: Quite simply, it's the loss of the ability to hear. It ranges in degree from the inability to detect quiet, high-pitched sound, to the inability to understand speech, to the inability to perceive any sound at all; the latter condition known as deafness.

Q: Is hearing loss common?

A: Yes. Approximately one in 10 Americans—more than 28 million—have some degree of hearing loss. And countless others—family members, friends and co-workers—are affected by this invisible condition, which has a profound impact on communication and daily life. The frustration of misunderstanding others and asking them to repeat themselves can leave people feeling lonely and isolated.

Q: But isn't hearing loss limited to older people?

A: No. Although a greater percentage of those who experience hearing loss are older, they are not the only ones. People of any age can lose their hearing.

Q: What causes hearing loss?

A: There are many causes, as we will discuss later. But to really understand these causes, you need to first understand the hearing process.

Q: Okay, how do we hear?

A: Hearing is a complicated process that involves the perception, conduction and interpretation of sound. The ear captures and translates sound waves into nerve impulses, which the brain receives and interprets.

Q: But the ear looks so simple. How can it do something so complicated?

A: Needless to say there's more to the ear than meets the eye. In fact, only part of the ear is visible. What we commonly call "the ear," the flesh-and-cartilage appendage known as the **auricle** or **pinna**, is simply a part of the **outer ear**.

Q: What are the other parts?

A: The outer ear consists of the pinna and the **ear canal**, which ends at the **tympanic membrane**, or **eardrum**. The eardrum forms the boundary between the outer ear and the **middle ear**, where the mechanics of hearing take place.

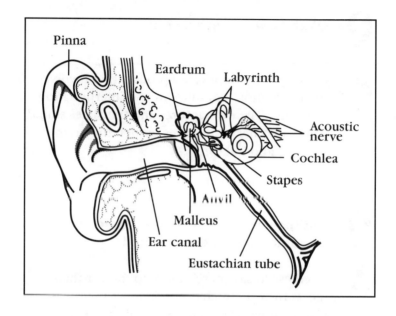

Pinna

Eardrum

Labyrinth

Acoustic nerve

Cochlea

Stapes

Anvil

Malleus

Ear canal

Eustachian tube

Q: **Would you explain those mechanics?**

A: Certainly. The pinna funnels sound waves into the ear canal, much like an old-fashioned ear trumpet funnels sound into the pinna. The ear canal then amplifies these sound waves and directs them to the eardrum. When the sound waves hit the eardrum, they set off vibrations that travel through three small bones called **ossicles**. You might remember their nicknames from health class—hammer, anvil and stirrup. These bones, also known as the **malleus**, **incus** and **stapes** respectively, vibrate in a chain reaction, conducting the sound waves through the middle ear. The innermost of these bones, the stapes, is the smallest bone in the body. When the stapes vibrates, it strikes a membrane called the **oval window**, propelling the sound waves through the membrane and into the **inner ear**.

Q: What happens in the inner ear?

A: That's where the sensory function of the hearing process takes place. The inner ear consists of two major parts—the **labyrinth** and the **cochlea**. The cochlea, which begins at the oval window and curves into a shape resembling a snail, acts much like a United Nations interpreter, translating sound from vibrations into electrical impulses that can be transmitted to the brain.

Q: How exactly does the cochlea work?

A: The cochlea is filled with fluid. Suspended in this fluid is the **basilar membrane**, a rubber-bandlike membrane attached at both ends to the walls of the cochlea. This membrane is covered with thousands of tiny hairs or **cilia**. At the base of these hairs are tiny nerve cells. When the stapes vibrates against the oval window, it causes the fluid and hairs to move. The movement of the hairs stimulates the nerve cells, which send the message, now in electronic-impulse form, to the brain via the **auditory nerve**, or **acoustic nerve**.

Q: You also mentioned the labyrinth. What is that?

A: The labyrinth is a group of three inter-connected, semicircular canals which controls our sense of balance.

Q: How does it do that?

A: Each canal is filled with fluid and is located at right angles to the other two. So whichever way you move your head, one or more of the canals detects the movement and relays the information to the brain.

Q: I didn't realize the ear was so complex. Are there any other parts I should be aware of?

A: Well, there is one other component—one you're probably aware of, at least indirectly. If you've ever had a cold that affected your ear or have blown your nose and felt your ear "pop," you probably realized that the ear is connected to the nose and throat in some way. That way is the **eustachian tube**, which directly links the middle ear to the oral cavity. The tube's role in hearing is to allow air to pass in and out of the middle ear, equalizing pressure on either side of the eardrum.

Q: Wow! Hearing is a very complicated process. What happens when there are problems?

A: A problem in any part of the ear can affect hearing if it impedes the conduction or interpretation of sound waves.

Let's go back to the path the sound waves must travel. They enter the ear through the pinna and are channeled through the ear canal.

Therefore, a deformed pinna or blocked ear canal could hinder the waves' progress to the eardrum and reduce hearing ability. If the waves reach the eardrum without a problem, but the eardrum is damaged, they may not be able to reach the ossicles. Likewise, any problem that prevents the ossicles from vibrating may prevent the sound waves from reaching the inner ear.

Once in the inner ear, the waves send ripples through the fluid to move the tiny hairs in the cochlea. Damage to the hairs or the nerve cells to which they are connected can affect the translation of the sound waves into electrical impulses. But even if the sound is translated correctly, the electrical impulses still must reach the brain. So, as you might guess, damage to the auditory nerve or the brain can also have a detrimental effect on hearing.

Q: **What causes these problems?**

A: There are many culprits and incidents, which we will discuss in detail later. But in general, these problems are caused by blockages or foreign objects in the ear, infections in the ear, diseases of the ear, diseases that secondarily affect the ear, injuries to the head, **ototoxic** drugs (i.e., toxic to the ear), changes in air pressure, noise exposure and the degeneration that occurs with aging. These causes comprise the two main types of hearing loss, which we'll discuss in detail in the next chapter.

2 LOSS CAUSES

Q: You said there are two major types of hearing loss?

A: Yes. Most hearing loss falls into one of two categories—conductive or sensorineural.

Conductive hearing loss occurs when the sound waves cannot be conducted from the outer or middle ear into the inner ear. A blockage in the ear canal, a punctured eardrum, a middle-ear infection or any problem that would prevent the eardrum or ossicles from vibrating produces a conductive loss.

Sensorineural hearing loss occurs either in the inner ear (the sensory part) or in the auditory nerve (the neural part). When sound reaches the inner ear but is not correctly perceived, or is correctly perceived but cannot reach the brain, the resulting loss is considered sensorineural. Damage to the hairs or nerve cells in the cochlea or damage to the auditory nerve produces a sensorineural loss.

Q: How can you tell which type of loss you have?

A: There are several factors that can clue you in. If your own voice sounds loud to you and other voices sound muffled, chances are your loss is conductive. Ringing in the ears, hearing better in noisy surroundings than in quiet surroundings, tolerating noises other people feel are too loud and speaking too softly for other people to hear are also characteristic of conductive loss.

If your voice sounds soft to you and you have difficulty understanding speech, you may have a sensorineural loss which is also known as nerve deafness. If you are sensitive to loud sounds, have difficulty hearing speech in noisy places and tend to speak in a loud voice, you probably have a sensorineural problem. Ringing or buzzing in the ears, a condition known as **tinnitus**, can also occur, but since this symptom is characteristic of both types of hearing loss, your best bet is to have your ears examined by a doctor.

Q: Can you have both types?

A: Yes. This is what is known as **mixed hearing loss**. It occurs when there are problems in both conduction and interpretation of sound. A loud explosion, for example, could puncture the eardrum and damage the hair cells in the cochlea, causing both conductive and sensorineural loss.

Q: Which hearing loss is more common?

A: Sensorineural loss is more common than conductive loss, primarily because aging-related hearing loss is sensorineural. Experts estimate that about 90 percent of all hearing loss is sensorineural.

Q: Which type is more serious?

A: Both types can be profound and can lead to deafness, but sensorineural loss is usually irreversible. Conductive loss, on the other hand, can often be reversed.

Q: That makes sense, since conductive loss is caused by something blocking the movement of the sound waves. You simply need to remove what's in the way, right?

A: Either that or repair the nonworking part that is stopping the sound waves. The reversal depends on the cause.

CAUSES AND PREVENTION OF CONDUCTIVE HEARING LOSS

Q: What are some of the causes of conductive loss?

A: Excessive earwax, foreign objects in the ear, **swimmer's ear**, surfer's ear, ruptured or perforated eardrums, ear infections, cysts, changes in air pressure or an abnormal bone growth known as **otosclerosis** can all give rise to conductive hearing loss. Fortunately, many of these problems can be remedied. A doctor can usually remove a foreign object from a person's ear without complications, for example, immediately reversing the hearing loss.

Q: I understand about foreign objects, but tell me more about how the other conditions cause hearing loss. Isn't earwax beneficial?

A: It is. Earwax or **cerumen** is produced in the ear canal to trap dust and other foreign particles before they can enter the more delicate parts of the ear. Normally, the ear produces just enough wax to do the job. In some instances, however, the ear produces too much wax. The excess wax hardens and blocks the ear canal. A blocked ear canal, of course, impedes sound waves and affects hearing.

Q: **Wouldn't regular ear cleaning prevent the problem?**

A: Not necessarily. In most cases, the ear cleans itself. Older wax usually makes its way to the opening of the ear canal, where it falls out or is washed away; meanwhile, newer wax is produced in the ear canal. Washing the outer ear with a washcloth can aid this process, but there is no need to regularly clean the ear canal. In fact, attempts to "clean" the ear with cotton swabs and other items may actually push the wax deeper into the ear and can damage the ear canal or eardrum. Your mother was right when she told you never to put anything smaller than an elbow in your ear.

Q: **So how can I get rid of excess wax?**

A: If you have a real wax problem—one that is affecting your hearing—you can try flushing your ear. This procedure does not involve sticking any foreign objects into the ear canal. To flush your ear, either assemble your own kit—some baby or mineral oil, an eyedropper and a syringe—or purchase a kit at the drugstore. If you buy a kit, follow the enclosed instructions. If you're a do-it-yourselfer, use the eyedropper to place a few drops of oil in your ear twice a day for several days (making sure you do not insert the dropper into the ear canal). This will soften the wax. Then, fill a bowl with body-temperature water, hold your head upright, pull your ear upward and squirt the water into your ear with the syringe, again making sure not to insert it into the ear canal. Turn your head and allow the water to drain out. You may have to repeat this flushing several times.

If the wax remains, visit your doctor. She, too, can flush the ear. She can also use suction or an instrument called a **curette** to scoop out the wax.

Q: Okay, I'll stay away from the cotton swabs. Maybe I should stay out of the water as well. How does swimmer's ear affect hearing?

A: Known officially as **otitis externa**, swimmer's ear is simply an inflammation of the outer ear canal. While it is often contracted through contact with water, it is not reserved for swimmers only. It can also occur when attempts to clean the ear with foreign objects irritate or tear the skin of the ear canal or allergies cause the ear canal to swell. The condition can be caused by a bacterial infection, a virus, an allergy or a fungus, and it usually includes eczema, a swelling of the skin. This swelling, which is often accompanied by itching, scaling and pain, can block the ear canal, affecting hearing.

Q: How can I get rid of swimmer's ear?

A: Since swimmer's ear is often caused by infection, you should see a doctor. Swimmer's ear is usually treated with corticosteroid eardrops and antibiotics. Corticosteroids (hormonal drugs) relieve the itching and reduce the inflammation. The antibiotics control the infection. Your role in the treatment, other than taking the medications, is to keep your ear dry so it will heal properly.

Q: Is there any way to prevent swimmer's ear?

A: There are several ways to reduce your risks of contracting it: Avoid swimming in polluted water, always dry your ears after bathing or swimming and avoid sticking foreign objects in your ear.

Q: What is surfer's ear, and how does it affect hearing?

A: Surfer's ear, also known as **exostosis**, is an abnormal bone growth in the ear canal. It is often triggered by exposure to cold water in the ear canal, which occurs when surfing. The growth blocks the ear canal and impedes the sound waves, affecting hearing. It is treated by surgically removing the growth.

Q: You also mentioned a ruptured eardrum. That could impede the sound waves' progress through the ossicles, right?

A: Right. A ruptured eardrum is a tear, perforation or hole in the eardrum. If you've ever tried to play a musical drum with a hole in its surface, you've heard how its power is diminished. The same thing happens to the eardrum. It still vibrates, but not as strongly, effectively reducing or stopping the sound waves' progress through the middle ear. In addition to hearing loss, a ruptured eardrum often produces pain and bleeding from the ear.

HAVE NOT EXPER. this though

Q: **What causes an eardrum to rupture?**

A: Cotton swabs, bobby pins and other small objects inserted far enough into the ear to puncture the eardrum are among the major culprits. Other causes include ear infections; head injuries; slaps on the ear; sudden changes in air pressure; and sudden, sharp, very loud noises, such as gunshots or explosions.

4th of July Fireworks

Q: **Can a ruptured eardrum heal?**

A: Yes. In most cases the eardrum will heal by itself as long it is kept dry and free from infection. Your doctor may prescribe an antibiotic to prevent or treat any infection. If the eardrum does not heal itself, your doctor can repair the tear with a tissue graft in a minor surgical procedure known as **tympanoplasty** or **myringoplasty**.

Q: The word infection has come up a lot. What causes infections and how can they get in the ear?

A: Infections can be caused by a variety of bacteria and viruses—from staphylococcus to herpes. These organisms, which make their way into your ears from outside or inside your body, settle in areas where the environment is conducive to their growth. In the case of swimmer's ear, for example, the presence of water or irritated skin creates this inviting environment.

Q: Where in the ear do infections occur?

A: Infections can occur anywhere throughout the ear and are usually referred to according to their location. Otitis externa, which we've already discussed, is an infection of the outer ear. Infections can also occur in the middle and inner ear. Middle-ear infections can affect hearing, while inner-ear infections can affect balance.

Q: I know ear infections are very common in children. Where do these infections occur and how common are they?

A: When people talk about ear infections, particularly children's ear infections, they're usually referring to infections of the middle ear.

Otitis media is the most common cause of conductive hearing loss and the most common cause of temporary hearing loss in young children, in whom it occurs most frequently. Approximately 80 percent of all children six and under have experienced at least one of these infections, which cost an estimated $3.5 billion annually to manage in the United States alone.

Q: What causes otitis media?

A: At the risk of sounding like a stuck record, there are many causes. Numerous bacteria and viruses can cause middle-ear infections, as can allergies, fungi or a dysfunctional eustachian tube. Anything that causes the eustachian tube to swell or be blocked, so that it provides inadequate ventilation into the middle ear, can cause an infection. And allergies, colds and other upper-respiratory infections can travel into the ears via the eustachian tube.

Q: No wonder it's so common! How serious is otitis media?

A: That depends. Middle-ear infections occur in several different forms and have many different causes. Definitely unpleasant, most produce pain, irritability and fever. **Otitis media with effusion**, an infection in which fluid accumulates in the middle ear, can also cause temporary hearing loss. As an added bonus, if fluid remains in the ear after the infection has gone, the infection may recur.

It is these recurring or chronic middle-ear infections, as well as infections that are left untreated, that prompt more serious problems. Untreated or uncontrolled otitis media can scar, thicken or rupture the eardrum, generate a cyst called **cholesteatoma**, lead to a bone infection known as **mastoiditis**, cause permanent hearing loss, and impair speech and language development in young children.

Q: Why does it hurt?

A: The pain is caused either by infected fluid in the middle ear pressing against the eardrum or by negative air pressure in the middle ear causing the eardrum to be sucked into the middle ear as if by a vacuum.

Q: What do you mean by negative air pressure?

A: Under normal circumstances, the eustachian tube equalizes the air pressure on both sides of the eardrum. When the tube becomes blocked or does not adequately ventilate the middle ear, the air pressure in the middle ear can drop.

Q: How does this affect hearing?

A: Anything that presses or pulls against the eardrum limits its mobility.

Q: Can anything be done for the pain?

A: Yes. While the infection itself requires a doctor's attention, you can relieve some of the pain by placing a warm heating pad on your ear and by taking aspirin or another pain reliever. Keep in mind, however, that children under 18 should not take aspirin because of its link to Reye's syndrome, an often fatal brain disease.

Q: How do doctors treat otitis media?

A: There are several treatment options, depending on the cause and type of infection. If the problem is caused by allergies, a cold or other congestion blocking the eustachian tube, your doctor may prescribe a decongestant or an antihistamine. To treat, control or prevent infection, however, antibiotics are the standard prescription.

Q: How effective are antibiotics in treating otitis media?

A: That is a matter of some debate. No antibiotic is effective for all ear infections all of the time, but there is evidence that some can be very successful in eradicating bacteria and relieving the pain in many cases.

Q: Can antibiotics prevent otitis media?

A: Evidence for their preventive abilities is mixed. A 1993 analysis of 27 studies on antibiotic treatment of otitis media published in the *Journal of the American Medical Association* found that antibiotics have beneficial but limited effect on preventing recurrent otitis media and limited short-term effect in treating otitis media with effusion. Still, the analysis found that antibiotics offer no real long-term benefit in treating otitis media with effusion. And we need to remember that no antibiotics are effective against viral infections.

Q: Which antibiotics are used to treat otitis media and how long are they used?

A: Because middle-ear infections have different causes, a variety of antibiotics is used. The most common is amoxicillin. Generally, the antibiotic is prescribed for about 10 days. Sometimes, however, the infection fails to clear up or recurs.

In these cases, doctors extend the use of the antibiotic. Long-term antibiotic use is common for treating stubborn infections or preventing future infections.

Q: I've heard there's some controversy about the long-term use of antibiotics for ear infections. What's the concern?

A: Actually, there are several. For one, the effectiveness is questionable, as we noted above. For another, long-term antibiotic use can cause side effects, such as diarrhea and skin rashes. The biggest concern, however, is the growing immunity of certain bacteria, including those which cause otitis media, to antibiotics.

Because of the widespread use of antibiotics, some bacteria have developed the ability to mutate to make themselves immune to certain antibiotics. As new antibiotics are tried, these stubborn bacteria continue their mutation and become immune to them as well. Eventually, these bacteria may become immune to all antibiotics, making it impossible to control infection.

Q: That sounds serious! Are there any other options available for treating otitis media?

A: Yes. Since antibiotics do not always work, particularly when the infection becomes chronic or involves persistent middle-ear fluid, a surgical procedure known as **myringotomy** can be performed or tubes can be placed in the ears.

Q: What is myringotomy?

A: Myringotomy is a procedure in which a small incision is made in the eardrum to relieve pressure or allow fluid to drain from the middle ear. As you recall, negative air pressure or fluid pressing against the eardrum causes the pain and hearing loss associated with otitis media. Creating a small opening in the eardrum relieves the pressure and allows the middle ear to drain. The eardrum then heals itself, usually within a day or two.

Q: That sounds simple, but what if the fluid returns after the eardrum recloses?

A: That's where the tubes come in. To assure that fluid can drain from the middle ear and air can enter the middle ear to equalize the pressure, a small plastic or metal tube is placed through the myringotomy incision, in effect creating a temporary eustachian tube. This procedure is called a **tympanostomy**.

Q: Is this procedure dangerous?

A: No surgical procedure is without risks. While tympanostomy can be done in either a doctor's office or in a hospital on an outpatient basis, it does usually require anesthesia. And, while the tympanostomy tubes can decrease the frequency and severity of middle-ear infections, thereby restoring hearing and preventing permanent hearing loss, there can be complications. Insertion can cause prolonged discharge from the ear, scar the eardrum or create a permanent hole in the eardrum. And the ear must be kept dry as long as the tubes are in, typically several months to a year.

Q: **There is a great deal of debate about putting tubes in children's ears. Why is it so controversial?**

A: For several reasons. While tympanostomy is not foolproof, it is often beneficial. It has the staunch support of the American Academy of Otolaryngology–Head and Neck Surgery, which represents the nation's ear specialists, and numerous pediatricians and other doctors, and is the most common operation performed on children in the United States (670,000 surgeries in 1988).

However, therein lies one of the concerns. The question is whether this common operation, like tonsillectomy, is always necessary or appropriate. And the answer varies depending on whom you ask. The debate heated up in April 1994, when a widely reported study that appeared in the *Journal of the American Medical Association* found that 23 percent of 6,611 recommendations for the tympanostomy tube insertions studied were inappropriate; 42 percent were appropriate and 35 percent were "equivocal," meaning their risks were equal to their benefits. Applying their findings

to the U.S. population in general, the authors
concluded that several hundred thousand
children each year may receive tubes that offer
them "no demonstrated advantage over less-
invasive therapies and may place them at
increased risk for undesirable outcomes." They
wrote that it is uncertain which patients benefit
from the tubes, and recommended that doctors
defer surgery for 90 days of watchful waiting.

Q: But you said most ear specialists support
this procedure?

A: They do. Their organization disputed the study,
claiming that it is prejudiced and inaccurate,
because it was not written by otolaryngologists
(ear specialists) and was done for use by health-
insurance companies. The Academy issued a
position statement indicating that watchful
waiting can allow bacteria to remain in the ear
and hearing to remain impaired. The statement
supports the use of tympanoplasty tubes, which
it said produce "immediate and satisfactory
results" and have been in part responsible for
the decrease in chronic ear disease and complications from otitis media over the last decade.

Q: Are there any other concerns about
ear tubes?

A: One more. It, too, is related to appropriateness.
Because tubes are usually not recommended
until a child has experienced ear infections for a

long time, often a period of years, he may actually outgrow the problem by the time the tubes are recommended.

Q: **These conflicting opinions don't help a parent decide whether he should let the doctor put tubes in his child's ears, do they?**

A: They sure don't. Until the medicos bring the debate to a close by coming up with a unified opinion, the best a parent can do is weigh the pros and cons of the procedure as it relates to his child. If her infection is recurrent, causes hearing loss and does not respond to antibiotics, tympanostomy may be the best bet. But as with any other controversial procedure, be sure to get an independent, second opinion.

Q: **I'm curious. What can happen if nothing is done for otitis media?**

A: The infection does go away on its own in many cases. In between 70 and 80 percent of children, the symptoms subside without treatment in one to three days. In others, however, the hearing loss becomes permanent and other complications arise.

Q: **What are these complications?**

A: The complications of uncontrolled otitis media include: inner-ear infection, which affects balance; development of a cholesteatoma; mastoiditis; brain abscess and meningitis.

Q: **Refresh my memory. What is a cholesteatoma?**

A: A cholesteatoma is a cyst in the middle ear. While it is relatively rare, it can cause hearing loss. Long-term negative air pressure in the middle ear, caused by eustachian-tube dysfunction or otitis media; growth of ear-canal skin through a ruptured eardrum, and growth of middle-ear skin are its primary causes.

A cholesteatoma blocks sound waves, causing conductive hearing loss. It can also erode the ossicles, resulting in permanent hearing loss. Left untreated, it can affect the facial nerve and cause meningitis. The only treatment for cholesteatoma is surgical removal. Reconstructive surgery can correct damage to the middle-ear bones, if necessary.

Q: **Okay. And mastoiditis is a bone infection, right?**

A: Right. When otitis media is left untreated, the infection can spread to the **mastoid** process, the bone behind the outer ear. This bone is connected to the middle ear. An infection of the mastoid process is known as mastoiditis, and can result in the destruction of the bone. Before antibiotics came on the scene, mastoiditis was a leading cause of death in children. Now, however, it is relatively rare. It can be treated with antibiotics or, in more stubborn cases, by the surgical removal of all or part of the mastoid bone, a procedure known as **mastoidectomy**.

Q: Let's get back to the other causes of conductive hearing loss. You mentioned a sudden change in air pressure. What is that called?

A: You're referring to **barotrauma**, a condition usually experienced while flying or scuba diving. These activities, which include sudden air-pressure changes, can cause earache, dizziness, a stuffy feeling in the ear and temporary hearing loss, especially when they are coupled with a blocked eustachian tube.

The symptoms are often enhanced by a cold or allergy and usually disappear within a few hours. But since they can be annoying, you might want to avoid them entirely. If you have a cold, try taking a decongestant or antihistamine before you fly and after you land; and during the flight, chew gum or suck on hard candy. If the symptoms persist long after your flight, see your physician. A myringotomy may be in order.

Q: You mentioned one other cause, otosclerosis. What is it and how does it cause hearing loss?

A: Otosclerosis, an abnormal growth of bone in the inner ear that affects the bones of the middle ear, is the most common cause of conductive hearing loss in young adults. Spongy bone begins to grow at the entrance to the inner ear, often immobilizing the stapes. When immobilized, the stapes cannot vibrate to pass sound waves into the inner ear, and a gradual, sometimes permanent, hearing loss develops.

Q: What causes otosclerosis?

A: No one knows for sure. But the disorder does seem to run in families. It is more common in women than in men, and in whites more than in African Americans, Native Americans or Asians. Normally slow and progressive, otosclerosis may increase in intensity and rate during pregnancy.

Q: Is there a cure?

A: There is no real cure for otosclerosis and no way to prevent it. There is, however, a surgical procedure that can often correct the damage caused by the disorder. And hearing aids may help in those cases where surgery is ineffective.

Q: Could you tell me about the surgery?

A: Certainly. The procedure is called a **stapedectomy**, because it involves the removal of the stapes. The tiny bone is either replaced entirely by a **prosthesis**, or only the footplate of the "stirrup" is replaced. The surgery results in temporary headache and dizziness and can, in rare cases, cause total hearing loss. Other possible complications include ear infection, development of a blood clot in the middle ear or rejection of the replacement. Usually, however, hearing improves quickly after the initial swelling from the surgery subsides.

CAUSES AND PREVENTION OF SENSORINEURAL HEARING LOSS

Q: What causes sensorineural hearing loss?

A: Remember, sensorineural loss affects the sensory and neural parts of the ear. It generally results from damage to the inner ear or damage to the auditory nerve. Anything that can cause this damage is a potential culprit, including: genetic or other congenital conditions, complications from various diseases, diseases or disorders of the ear, head injury or trauma, exposure to ototoxic drugs, noise exposure and aging.

Q: Sensorineural loss is usually irreversible, right?

A: Right. But don't panic. There are varying levels of hearing loss, not all of which are handicapping, and a number of devices on the market make it easier to cope with a serious hearing loss.

Q: That's somewhat reassuring. Not all of the causes are as common as the last two, are they?

A: No. But they shouldn't be discounted. While they affect a smaller percentage of the population, they can be just as, if not more, serious. Some of these conditions are among the primary causes of infant and childhood deafness, and others are accompanied by a number of complications.

Q: I assume it's the congenital and genetic disorders that affect the youngsters?

A: You assume correctly. The various genetic disorders together form one of if not *the* major cause of sensorineural loss in children. In fact, experts estimate that genetic disorders are responsible for at least half of all **profound** deafness in childhood. And other, nongenetic congenital conditions—those present at birth— can also result in deafness.

Q: What are some of these disorders and conditions?

A: Among the most common of the genetic disorders are Usher's syndrome, which occurs in between 3 and 10 percent of patients with congenital deafness; Waardenburg's syndrome, which occurs in 1 to 2 percent, and Alport's syndrome, which occurs in approximately 1 percent. Causes of congenital hearing loss other than genetic disorders include: prematurity, neonatal jaundice, cerebral palsy, hypothyroidism, quinine intoxication, syphilis, prenatal exposure to drugs such as thalidomide or tretinoin and prenatal exposure to viral infections such as rubella (German measles) or chicken pox.

Q: A number of those are disease-related. What diseases cause sensorineural hearing loss later in life?

A: Glad you asked. Sensorineural loss is a complication of a number of ailments: syphilis, in which the bacteria invade the inner ear and damage the cochlea and auditory nerve; tuberculosis, which perforates the eardrum as well as causes sensorineural damage; bacterial meningitis, which damages the hair cells or auditory nerve, causing hearing loss in between 5 and 35 percent of its survivors; multiple sclerosis, leukemia and autoimmune disorders like lupus, which can swell blood vessels in the ear; circulatory disorders, which affect circulation in the inner ear and can cause hemorrhaging; viral infections, such as mumps, scarlet fever, herpes, rubella, chicken pox, mononucleosis and pertussis; diabetes; and tumors of the inner ear or auditory nerve.

Q: **You can get a tumor in your ear?**

A: You sure can. Cancer can spread into the ear, and noncancerous, or benign, tumors can also develop. Tumors of the **temporal bone**, a large bone on either side of the head of which the mastoid is a part, also affect hearing. If the tumor invades the outer or middle ear, it produces conductive loss; if it affects the inner ear or auditory nerve, it produces sensorineural loss.

Q: **How serious is a tumor?**

A: That depends on the type and where it's located. Obviously, a cancerous tumor poses a health risk. And even noncancerous tumors can damage surrounding parts as they grow. For example, **acoustic neuroma**, a commonly occurring noncancerous tumor of the auditory or acoustic nerve, can create pressure on various vital brain structures and damage them.

Q: Can anything be done about these tumors?

A: The only treatment is surgical removal, which stops the growth of the tumor and its progressive damage. In some cases, surgical removal of acoustic neuroma also restores some of the lost hearing ability.

Q: Getting back to the other causes, you said there are disorders or diseases of the ear?

A: Yes. We've already talked about a few of them—otosclerosis and other genetic disorders, for example. There is one more we need to discuss: **Ménière's disease**.

Q: What is that?

A: Ménière's disease is a chronic illness that comes and goes in unpredictable attacks. Excess fluid builds up in the inner ear, causing fluctuating hearing loss, tinnitus and intense periods of dizziness or **vertigo**, which are often accompanied by nausea and vomiting.

Q: What causes the fluid to build up?

A: No one knows. Some experts speculate that allergies, viruses, infections and head injuries may be in some way responsible.

Q: Who is most susceptible to Ménière's disease?

A: The disorder can affect anyone at any age, but it is most common in people between the ages of 30 and 60. And it affects women more often than men.

Q: Is there any cure?

A: No cure, but there are treatments. Your doctor can give you medication to control the dizziness and nausea. And diuretics, a low-salt diet and a reduction in caffeine and alcohol consumption are often recommended to decrease fluid in the body.

In instances where the vertigo is severe, surgery may be recommended. There are several types—an operation that opens the labyrinth to allow excess fluid to drain out; one which severs the nerve that controls balance; or **labyrinthectomy**, the removal of the entire inner ear. The latter, of course, destroys all hearing in the ear.

Q: Why would anyone resort to such a drastic procedure?

A: In some instances, the dizziness associated with Ménière's disease is so severe it debilitates. This last-resort procedure alleviates the problem. Labyrinthectomy is usually reserved for people who have lost all or almost all of the hearing in the affected ear and retain hearing ability in the other ear.

Q: Back to other causes. How can trauma affect hearing?

A: Trauma caused by a sudden physical change or injury, can affect the hearing in a number of ways. Remember, a sudden blow to the head can cause the eardrum to rupture, and a sudden change in air pressure can produce barotrauma, causing conductive hearing loss.

Trauma can also cause sensorineural hearing loss. Fractures to the skull or injuries that cause concussion can damage the cochlea or auditory nerve. And recent evidence suggests that even the jarring caused by high-impact aerobics may damage the hair cells of the cochlea, resulting in sensorineural hearing loss.

Q: What are the most common causes of trauma?

A: A blow to the ear, sudden loud noises like explosions or gunfire, and long-term exposure

to loud noise are the most common causes of
acoustic trauma.

Q: I take it there's no cure for hearing loss caused by trauma?

A: Not if the loss is sensorineural in nature. Remember, a perforated eardrum can be repaired, but cochlear hair cells cannot. Hearing aids and other listening devices or techniques are the only treatment for this type of hearing loss. We'll discuss these tools, the effects of noise exposure and how to prevent hearing loss from noise exposure in more detail later.

Q: Well, I'd like some preventive advice right now. You mentioned that certain drugs can cause sensorineural hearing loss. Could you tell me what they are, so I can avoid them?

A: A number of commonly used drugs are toxic to the ear and can cause tinnitus and hearing loss. The majority do this by damaging the hair cells in the cochlea. Among the most common: aspirin and other salicylates; aminoglycoside antibiotics, including amikacin, neomycin, kanamycin, streptomycin and gentamicin; the antibiotics vancomycin and erythromycin; loop diuretics such as ethracrynic acid and furosemide; and quinine and antineoplastic agents such as the cancer drug cisplatin.

Q: Does this mean I should never take these drugs?

A: Not at all. These are side effects that may or may not occur depending on your condition, the dosage and the other drugs you may be taking. For example, patients with kidney failure are more likely to experience hearing loss from aminoglycoside antibiotics than are other patients. You and your doctor need to be aware of the possibility of ototoxicity. If your doctor prescribes an ototoxic drug, he should check with you periodically to make sure that you are not experiencing hearing loss. Let him know right away if a problem arises. And if you experience tinnitus or hearing loss when taking aspirin, stop taking it and notify your doctor.

Q: Will the problem go away if I stop taking the ototoxic drug?

A: That depends on the drug in question. Hearing loss caused by certain ototoxic drugs, like aspirin or erythromycin, usually reverses itself after the drug is discontinued. And in nearly all cases, the progression of hearing loss will stop with discontinuation. Remember, however, that most of these drugs damage hair cells in the cochlea. And hair cells cannot be replaced. If serious damage has been done, hearing loss will be permanent. That's why it's important to notify your doctor immediately if you have any problems.

Q: You keep mentioning those hair cells. I know they're important and I assume they're pretty delicate, but what kind of damage are you talking about?

A: The hair cells, whose movement inside the cochlea sends messages to the nerve cells, are indeed delicate, and they can be damaged just like any other hairs. Rather than just inconveniencing their owner with the embarrassment of split ends, however, these hairs die and do not grow back. Their cause of death can usually be attributed to illness, noise or aging.

Q: Is there any hope on the horizon for hair cells? Anything like minoxidil?

A: Retinoic acid, the vitamin A derivative used to prevent skin from aging, may be an answer. Scientists at the Albert Einstein College of Medicine in New York and the University of Liege in Belgium used retinoic acid on the hair cells of rats and found that up to 78 percent of the hair cells were regenerated. Of course, research must still determine whether retinoic acid will have a similar effect on human hair cells.

Q: So much for illness; now to noise. It seems ironic that noise—what you hear—can cause hearing loss. Is all noise a problem?

A: Generally, only sudden, very loud noise or prolonged exposure to loud noise causes serious damage to hair cells. We already discussed how sudden loud noises, such as explosions or gunfire, can cause acoustic trauma. But long-term exposure can also be a problem.

Have you ever been at a loud concert or sporting event for several hours, then had difficulty hearing conversation when you left the stadium? The condition probably became less and less noticeable until things finally sounded normal again. This is what is called a **temporary threshold shift**. Your hair cells changed temporarily in response to the noise, and as a result, your hearing sensitivity, or threshold, also changed.

Repeated exposure to loud noise, however, can produce a **permanent threshold shift**. In this case, the hair cells change permanently, resulting in a permanent change in your sensitivity to sound.

Q: What do you mean by loud?

A: That's a good question. Most people rate loudness in a relative way. Rock music that a teenager might term normal might seem extremely loud to an adult. To determine loudness in a more objective, standardized fashion, a unit of measure called the **decibel** was developed. Generally, any noise that is 90 decibels or more can damage your ear if you're exposed to it for a long period of time.

Q: But what does that mean? How loud is a decibel?

A: While a decibel is a standardized measure, it is also a relative measure. To put it in perspective, a large truck, motorcycle, city traffic or a table saw generates noise near the 90-decibel level. A portable stereo with headphones at half-volume measures between 100 and 110 decibels. And jet-engine noise measures about 130 decibels. Average conversation, on the other hand, is generally around 60 decibels.

Remember, the decibel is a relative unit of measure. It is based on a logarithmic scale measured in 10s. Literally, a decibel (named after telephone inventor Alexander Graham Bell) is one-tenth of a bel. A noise that is 20 decibels is 10 times louder than a 10-decibel noise. Thus, noise that is 90 decibels is many times louder than normal conversation. No wonder it can damage our ears!

Q: How long must you be exposed to the noise before it begins to affect your hearing?

A: That depends on the level of noise. In some instances, your hearing can be damaged in a matter of seconds. The general rule is: Exposure to noise levels of 90 decibels or more should be limited. You should be exposed to no more than eight hours a day of 90-decibel noise; four hours a day of 95-decibel noise; two hours a day of 100-decibel noise; one hour a day of 105-decibel noise; 30 minutes a day of 110-decibel noise and

15 minutes a day of 115-decibel noise or your hearing can be affected. Noise above 115 decibels is not considered safe for any length of time.

Q: **But what if you can't limit the exposure? What if the noise is job-related?**

A: Occupational hearing loss is a real problem. Of the more than 20 million Americans who are exposed to dangerous levels of noise on a daily basis, 9 million are exposed on the job. There is, however, a law to protect workers. The Occupational Safety and Health Administration (OSHA) requires employers to protect their employees from extended noise levels of 85 decibels and above. If you work in a loud environment without noise control or hearing protection, talk to your employer and ask him to comply with the OSHA standards. If he refuses, contact your local OSHA office.

Q: **What type of hearing protection is available?**

A: There are two basic types of hearing-protection devices: **earplugs** and **earmuffs**. Earplugs are used to protect against low-frequency or low-pitched sounds, while muffs are usually used to protect against high-frequency, or high-pitched, sounds. Most can usually reduce the noise level between 15 and 30 decibels. When worn together, the noise level can drop an additional 10 to 15 decibels.

Q: Which protects better, earplugs or earmuffs?

A: That depends on the product and your needs. There are different varieties of both, and their effectiveness varies. All are labeled with a noise-reduction rating (NRR) that estimates the reduction in decibels reaching your ear. An NRR of 20, for example, indicates that, when wearing the device, the sound level actually reaching your ear will be 20 decibels less than the sound level around you. The best protection is afforded by devices that have an NRR of 30 or higher.

Q: Tell me more about earplugs. Are you talking about those little rubber things you buy at the drugstore?

A: Those and others, yes. Inexpensive, disposable earplugs do protect against noise exposure. But they are not the only type of earplugs available. Earplugs can be disposable and nondisposable; bought over the counter or custom fitted. They can be made of rubber, sponge, foam rubber, silicone, acrylic, vinyl, wax-impregnated cotton and other materials.

The over-the-counter earplugs work by being inserted into the ear canal, and by either conforming to the anatomy of the canal or expanding to fit the canal. Custom-made earplugs are custom-fitted to your ear. These earplugs can also be modified by adding filters, vents and other features that can further protect hearing.

Q: **How about earmuffs? Don't they merely keep your ears warm?**

A: They might, but you're talking about a whole different species. The earmuffs we're interested in are not the soft, fuzzy cloth contraptions that people drape over their heads each winter. These muffs, worn either with a band over the head, behind the head or under the chin, or attached to a helmet, look more like earphones. Made of rubber, metal, plastic or other materials, they have cushions that are filled with a sound-absorbent material such as foam or liquid. These muffs must fit snugly around your ear to be most effective.

Q: **Are there any other ways to protect yourself from noise exposure?**

A: Certainly, although all may not be appropriate in every case. Obviously, it is most important to limit your exposure to loud noises whenever possible. Make sure the volume on your television or stereo is at a reasonable level, particularly if it's a personal stereo or you're using headphones. If your leisure activities are loud, limit your participation. Avoid buying loud appliances or toys. And be aware of the noise level around you. If you have to shout to make yourself heard, the noise level is probably too loud.

Q: Most older people have had lots of exposure to noise. Is that one of the reasons for age-related hearing loss?

A: It sure is. The long-term effects of noise on the hair cells, as well as the death of hair cells due to other causes—including, in some cases, a decreased blood supply to the ear caused by heart disease or high blood pressure, heredity and simple deterioration with age—are the major reasons for age-related hearing loss, which is also known as **presbycusis**.

Q: How common is presbycusis?

A: Extremely common. In fact, it is the greatest cause of hearing impairment in adults. Estimates vary, but approximately 30 percent of all Americans over 65 have some degree of hearing loss. And that percentage increases with age. By some counts, 50 percent of those 75 or older suffer from presbycusis. And with our longevity increasing and millions of baby boomers hitting middle age, the number of people with age-related hearing loss is bound to increase dramatically.

Q: Does presbycusis come on suddenly?

A: No. It's a gradual process, often beginning between the ages of 40 and 50. Usually, it starts

with difficulty hearing high-pitched sounds.
In some instances, the loss is so minor it goes
unnoticed. In others, it gradually worsens until
it becomes quite severe.

Q: **Who is more affected by presbycusis?
Men or women?**

A: Sorry, guys. Men are affected more commonly
and more severely than women.

Q: **I think you answered this before, but is
there any cure for presbycusis?**

A: No. Once the cochlea is damaged, the hearing
loss is permanent. There are, however, ways to
cope and adapt with the loss, including **speech
reading**, **assistive listening devices** and
adaptive equipment for household use. We'll
discuss these later.

3 TESTING. ONE...TWO...THREE...

Q: I think I might be losing my hearing. Could you review some of the symptoms?

A: Certainly. If you are told you speak either too loudly or too softly; if you hear better in noisy surroundings or have difficulty hearing speech in noisy surroundings; if you have difficulty understanding women's and children's voices or other high-pitched sounds; if you are able to tolerate sounds others say are too loud; if you must often ask others to repeat what they have said or you find yourself misunderstanding speech or watching people more carefully when they speak; if you play the radio or television at a loud volume; if you have pain or discharge from your ear or if you suffer from dizziness or tinnitus, you may have some degree of hearing loss. If you are older and suspect you have hearing loss, a brief questionnaire in Appendix A may help you determine whether you have symptoms of presbycusis.

Q: What about infants and young children? How can you tell if they might have hearing loss?

A: Good question. While hearing loss is more common among adults than children, some 3 million American children do have a hearing loss. And experts estimate that slightly more than one-third of these children are under three years of age. Obviously, these children may not be able to recognize or tell you about their symptoms—especially if their hearing loss has affected their language development—so you need to recognize these signs on your own.

Q: What are some of the signs?

A: Within the first six months, the infant should react in some way to unexpected loud noises, imitate sounds and turn his head in the direction of a familiar voice. Moving on through his first year, he should be able to babble, point to familiar people or objects when asked and understand simple phrases. And between his first and second year, he should respond when called, respond to sounds, locate where sound is coming from, begin to use simple words, and show growth in understanding and using words to communicate. If your child fails to develop these behaviors, he may have a hearing problem and should see a doctor. For a more complete listing of possible problems, see Appendix B.

Q: Can a young child's hearing be tested?

A: Yes, it can. In fact, a National Institutes of Health panel recently recommended that all newborns have their hearing screened before they leave the hospital or at least sometime within their first three months. Early screening, primarily through the use of computerized tests that measure the function of the inner ear and auditory nerve, leads to earlier detection of hearing problems, and perhaps fewer language development problems. Without early screening, hearing problems usually are not detected until a child is between one and three years old— a crucial age for language development.

Q: Back to adults. Is testing the first thing I should have done if I suspect I'm losing my hearing?

A: It's certainly an important step, but it should not be the first. Remember, hearing loss has a number of causes, and could be a symptom of other medical problems. Your first step is to schedule an examination with your family doctor. He should review your medical history, ask you questions about your hearing loss and other conditions or symptoms and examine your ears with an **otoscope**.

Q: What's that?

A: The otoscope, or otomicroscope, is a small microscope. It is often attached to a speculum, a hollow, funnel-shaped instrument that fits into the ear canal. A pneumatic otoscope also has a rubber tube attached to a small rubber bulb, which enables the doctor to change the air pressure in the ear.

Q: Why do that?

A: Remember, a healthy eardrum is mobile. It should move back and forth as air pressure in the ear changes. If the eardrum does not move, it could indicate a problem—perhaps a buildup of fluid in the middle ear or negative air pressure in the middle ear.

Q: Does the doctor actually see the eardrum with the otoscope?

A: Yes. He can see and examine both the eardrum and the ear canal. And with the pneumatic otoscope, he can also test the mobility of the eardrum.

Q: **Are there any other tools doctors can use to examine the ear?**

A: Yes, there are. Two other commonly used instruments are the **acoustic otoscope** and the **tympanometer**, both of which can detect fluid in the middle ear. The acoustic otoscope reflects sound waves off the eardrum; while the tympanometer sends a tone through the ear and measures how much of it is absorbed by the eardrum.

Q: **Will the doctor do anything other than examine my ear?**

A: He may perform some diagnostic tests to determine the location and cause of your hearing loss. We'll discuss these hearing tests later on.

Q: **What happens after the examination?**

A: That depends on what the doctor discovers. If the doctor finds that excess wax has caused your problem, for example, he may flush out your ear. If the examination reveals that you have one of the many ailments of which hearing loss is a complication, you may be treated for that condition. And if your doctor cannot determine the cause of your hearing loss, finds that it is beyond the scope of his treatment ability or believes you may benefit from a hearing aid, he may suggest that you see a specialist.

Q: What kind of specialists are there?

A: The medical doctor whose specialty includes the ear is called an **otolaryngologist**. These doctors, formerly called **otorhinolaryngologists**, are also known as ear, nose and throat specialists or **ENT**s, because they specialize in treating the ears, nose, throat and related structures of the head and neck. Otolaryngologists who sub-specialize in the ear are called **otologists**.

Q: What can an otolaryngologist do?

A: Otolaryngologists can examine, diagnose, treat and manage injuries and disorders of the ear, as well as the nose, throat, face, jaws and other areas of the head and neck. They are trained to perform surgery, including ear operations, such as tympanostomy, myringotomy and tumor removal. They can also perform cosmetic facial plastic surgery, treat cancer of the head and neck, and treat allergic, sinus, laryngeal, thyroid and esophageal disorders.

Q: What kind of training do they have?

A: Otolaryngologists are doctors who have com-pleted medical school, received their M.D. or D.O. degree, then pursued five years of post-graduate specialty training under supervision (called a residency). Their training must include one or more years of general surgery and three or more years of otolaryngology—head-and-neck-surgery training in an approved residency program. After they have completed this training and passed a written examination, they can be certified by the American Board of Otolaryngology.

Q: What do you mean by certified?

A: The purpose of certification, according to the American Board of Medical Specialties, is to "provide assurance to the public that a certified medical specialist has successfully completed an approved educational program and an evaluation ... designed to assess the knowledge, experience and skills requisite to the provision of high-quality patient care in that specialty."

Essentially, passing the board-certification exam means that a doctor has been deemed worthy by his peers of practicing in his specialty. A board-certified specialist is likely to be competent in his field.

Q: Can an otologist be certified as well?

A: Yes. An otolaryngologist can receive subspecialty certification in otology/neurotology. This means he has completed at least one year of additional training in the diagnosis, management, prevention, cure and care of patients with disease of the ear and temporal bone, including disorders of hearing and balance. This training is usually in the form of a fellowship.

Q: Are there any other subspecialties of otolaryngology?

A: There is one other—pediatric otolaryngology. A pediatric otolaryngologist, obviously, specializes in treating children. He has special expertise in congenital and acquired conditions involving the ear and skills in managing childhood disorders of voice, speech, language and hearing.

Q: Do any other professionals deal with hearing loss?

A: Yes. **Audiologists** also specialize in hearing loss. These allied health professionals are trained to measure hearing loss and rehabilitate people with communication problems. They often work in tandem with otolaryngologists, administering hearing tests and assisting the hearing impaired with listening devices and coping strategies.

Q: What type of training do they have?

A: While the term audiologist has been used by some unscrupulous hearing-aid companies to refer to their untrained dealers, true audiologists must receive formal training at the graduate level and put in hours of clinical practice. The majority of states require them to be licensed, and most are certified by the American Speech-Language-Hearing Association. To be certified and receive the Certificate of Clinical Competence in Audiology (CCC-A), an audiologist must have a graduate degree in audiology or speech-language pathology, complete 350 hours of clinical experience and pass a rigorous exam. Only certified audiologists can place the letters CCC-A after their names.

Q: **You mentioned hearing-aid dealers. What do they do?**

A: Hearing-aid dealers sell, fit and service hearing aids. In many cases, they also perform hearing tests.

Q: **Do they have any training?**

A: Some do and some don't. Many audiologists are hearing-aid dealers, for example. But other dealers may simply be salespeople. There is no specific training required by the federal government to dispense hearing aids, and state training-and-licensing requirements vary. Some states do require dealers to undergo an apprenticeship program before they can be licensed, and many reputable companies train their staffs to test hearing and fit hearing aids. In addition, the International Hearing Society, formerly the National Hearing Aid Society, a nonprofit trade organization, offers continuing education courses and a voluntary certification program for hearing-aid dealers through its National Board for Certification of Hearing Instrument Sciences (BC-HIS). Dealers who have been certified can include the letters BC-HIS in their titles. Since the training and licensing vary so greatly, it is wise to ask any dealer who is not a certified audiologist what his credentials are.

Q: **We're jumping the gun here. I'm not ready to see a hearing-aid dealer yet. What's the next step after the medical exam?**

A: After your family doctor or an ear specialist has examined your ears, he will probably suggest that you have your hearing evaluated. This information, which in some cases helps pinpoint the cause of the problem, is essential in determining how your hearing loss should be treated.

Q: **Where should I go to get my hearing tested?**

A: That depends. If your ear specialist does hearing testing or works in conjunction with an audiologist, you can probably get your hearing tested right at his office. If he does not test, ask him to refer you to an independent, certified audiologist.

Q: Couldn't I just go to a hearing-aid dealer? The one in my town offers free hearing tests.

A: Remember, training-and-licensing requirements for hearing-aid dealers vary from state to state. There is no easy way to guarantee that the dealer you visit is adequately trained and competent in hearing assessment. You need to remember that a hearing-aid dealer's primary role is to sell hearing aids. The free test may be simply a gimmick to lure you into his showroom, and until you've had your hearing evaluated by a qualified examiner, you don't know whether or not you will benefit from a hearing aid.

Q: Understood. What can I expect from a hearing evaluation?

A: A hearing evaluation, no matter whom it is performed by, will probably include a variety of tests. Among the possibilities are tests to determine: whether the hearing loss is stronger in one ear than the other; whether the hearing loss is conductive or sensorineural; at what pitch the hearing loss begins; at what loudness level the hearing loss begins; and what words and sounds can and cannot be distinguished.

Q: How many of these tests will be done?

A: The exact number and type of tests you will undergo depends on what is already known about your hearing problem and whether a hearing aid is a recommended option. But tests to determine the pitch and loudness at which your hearing loss begins and your ability to understand speech are standard in almost every hearing evaluation.

Q: **Didn't you say some of these tests might be done at the initial medical exam?**

A: They can be. Tests to determine the location and type of hearing loss, for example, are often done during the initial medical exam, and other diagnostic tests might be performed at the initial exam or the specialist's exam. Obviously, the goal of these tests is to find the cause of your hearing problem. If the cause is treatable, treatment is probably the next option. If it is not, your actual ability to hear will be tested.

Q: **You said these diagnostic tests can determine whether hearing loss is stronger in one ear than another. Is that possible?**

A: Because most hearing loss is sensorineural, most hearing loss occurs in both ears, or is **bilateral**. The loss can, however, be stronger in one ear than in the other. One ear may have been exposed to more noise, for example, or experienced more ear infections. Hearing loss, particularly the conductive type, can also be **unilateral**, meaning it occurs in only one ear. With this in mind, tests to determine the relative strength and location of hearing loss are usually among the first performed, if they are needed.

Q: What tests are used?

A: The tests used to determine the strength and location of hearing loss are among the simplest in the hearing evaluation; they use a old-fashioned tuning fork, rather than high-tech gadgetry and tools. A vibrating tuning fork is placed first near one ear and then near the other, and the person is asked in which ear she heard the sound better. If she is unsure, the doctor may perform **Weber's test**. In this test, the vibrating fork is placed on the patient's forehead, nose bridge or chin, and she is asked in which ear she hears better. The results are immediate and obvious.

Q: Can the tuning fork be used for any other tests?

A: It sure can. A third tuning-fork test, the **Rinne test**, determines the nature of the hearing loss. In this test, the vibrating fork is held near one ear, first in the air and then with its stem against the mastoid bone behind the ear. Someone who hears the sound louder through the ear either has normal hearing or a sensorineural loss. Someone who hears the sound louder through bone has a conductive loss. This test, too, produces immediate, obvious results.

Q: What other diagnostic tests can be used either at the exam or in a hearing evaluation?

A: If the cause of your hearing problem is still unknown, but the doctor has some idea where the problem is located, several additional tests may be helpful. The tympanometer can be used to gather information about the function of the eardrum or middle ear; **electrocochleography** can be used to gain information about the inner ear; and **brain stem audiometry** can provide information about the function of the hearing centers of the brain. The latter two tests involve placing electrodes at specific spots to record the ear or brain's response to sound.

Q: I thought the only tests done used headphones. What do those headphone tests measure anyway?

A: The tests you're probably most familiar with— the **pure-tone audiometry** tests, which often use headphones—are the ones that determine at what level you hear specific **frequencies**, or pitches. In these tests, which are a standard part of any hearing evaluation, you either put on a pair of headphones or have a vibrating device placed on the mastoid bone behind your ear. The headphones or vibrator is connected to an instrument called an **audiometer**, which produces sounds of different frequencies and intensities. Your job is to signal when you hear the tone. The softest level at which you hear the

sound—your **pure-tone threshold**—is then
plotted on a graph called an **audiogram**.

Q: What exactly does this graph tell you?

A: The audiogram tells you at what loudness level
or intensity you hear certain frequencies.

Q: I can understand why you'd want to know
how loud something has to be for you to
hear it, but why would you need to know
anything about frequencies?

A: Primarily because certain sounds occur only at
certain frequencies. Let's back up a minute. We
defined frequency as pitch—something we can
identify with. But in reality, a frequency is the
speed at which the sound waves travel. It is
measured in the number of cycles per second or
Hertz (abbreviated Hz). If a sound travels slowly,
it has a low number of cycles per second and a
low pitch. If it travels quickly, it has a high
number of Hertz and a high pitch.

Getting back to your question, a normal ear
has the ability to hear sound in frequencies
between 20 and 20,000 Hz. Normal human
speech occurs between 500 and 2,000 Hz, with
the vowels falling below 1,000 Hz and the
consonants above 1,000 Hz. So a hearing loss in
the frequencies between 1,000 and 2,000 Hz
would affect the way you understand speech.
You would not hear specific consonants; you

might mistake one word for another or not hear
certain words at all. So, as you can see, identi-
fying the frequencies you can and cannot hear
helps the professionals understand and correct
the handicaps you may be experiencing as a
result of hearing loss.

Q: **Couldn't they just ask you what sounds
you hear?**

A: They could, but many people are not aware of
their problem, and others deny they have a problem. There are, however, some simple **speech-
discrimination tests** that are performed to
determine exactly which sounds you do and do
not hear.

Q: **Could you explain these tests?**

A: Of course. Speech-discrimination tests, the other
standard tests in hearing evaluations, measure
how accurately you distinguish the sounds of
speech in words. The person doing the testing
speaks to you through a pair of earphones, pro-
nouncing various words, which you are asked
to repeat. If you're having trouble distinguishing
between certain consonants or vowels, the
problem will become obvious.

Q: **That sounds simple. Are there any other kinds of speech tests?**

A: Yes. A similar test can be performed to see at what level you can distinguish certain sounds. Again, you are asked to repeat words spoken to you through earphones. In this instance, however, the tester varies the loudness of the words you hear.

Q: **Wow! I didn't know there were so many kinds of hearing tests out there. What happens after I've had the ones I need?**

A: That depends on the tests. As we've already discussed, results of diagnostic tests may lead to other diagnostic tests, possible treatment for the cause of your hearing loss, or if the hearing loss is permanent, speech and audiometry testing. After the speech and audiometry tests, you will be told at what decibel level you hear specific frequencies.

Q: **Won't the tester tell me what percent of hearing loss I have?**

A: She may, but it doesn't mean very much. Percent of hearing loss, a figure derived based on a complicated formula, was designed primarily to be used in a legal setting to determine how much compensation a person with hearing loss should receive from the party who caused the loss. The figure, which is calculated based on decibels lost multiplied by a formula that yields a percentage, is appropriate for this legal use, as it ranks hearing loss across the board and gives a general result that can be easily understood. But it is not an accurate representation of hearing loss.

Q: Why not?

A: The problem with this figure is that it fails to take into account the fact that you can have different amounts of hearing loss in different frequencies. To say someone has 40 percent hearing loss doesn't tell you, for example, whether or not that person has difficulty hearing low pitches.

Q: So how is hearing measured?

A: By decibels and frequencies. You can, for example, have a 20-decibel loss in higher frequencies and no loss in lower frequencies. This would mean you may have difficulty hearing high-pitched sounds, but no problem at all hearing sounds in lower registers.

Q: **That is a more specific way of measuring. But how do I know how severe my loss is?**

A: Basically, you use that same information and apply it to some generalized rules. A loss of between 0 and 20 decibels is considered minor; a 20- to 40-decibel loss is moderate; a 65- to 70-decibel loss is severe and a loss of 90 or more decibels is profound (nearing deafness).

Q: **I understand the ranking, but it's hard for me to judge what a 60-decibel loss would be. Could you put this in a different perspective?**

A: Certainly. A 60-decibel loss would mean that you hear no sounds in that frequency below 60 decibels. Remember, 60 decibels is the average level of conversation. So a person with a 60-decibel loss would have great difficulty hearing conversation in that frequency, but would have no trouble hearing, say a chain saw.

Q: **I see. But how is that information used?**

A: Primarily to determine what, if any kind of corrective action can be taken. If the hearing loss is mild, for example, you may simply be advised of the problem and taught a few coping skills. Hearing aids and/or assistive-listening devices may be recommended for more severe loss. The measurements help determine what type of hearing aid may provide the most benefit, something we'll examine in detail in the next chapter.

4 HEARING AIDS AND OTHER DEVICES

HEARING AIDS

Q: What if a hearing aid is recommended for me? Will that restore my hearing?

A: No. Hearing aids can improve but not restore your sensory ability.

Q: How do they improve hearing?

A: Hearing aids amplify sound and can be tuned to amplify the frequencies where the loss is greatest. They cannot, however, compensate for all speech distortions or restore your sensitivity to sound in every frequency.

Q: You mean speech may still sound distorted, even with a hearing aid?

A: Yes. Speech distortion occurs when you cannot hear certain sounds used in speech, so the words sound incomplete and distorted. Failure to understand high-frequency consonant sounds such as s or th, for example, would make the words "sing" and "thing" indistinguishable. Both would sound like "ing," a distortion of the intended word. Combine that with hundreds of other distorted words, and speech becomes very difficult to understand.

A hearing aid can compensate for many of these distortions by amplifying sounds in the frequencies in which they occur. But it may not be able to amplify all of the frequencies to the level at which you begin to hear them. You may still have gaps in what you hear. Certain sounds may still be undetectable, so speech may continue to sound incomplete or distorted. In addition, other sounds in the amplified frequencies may seem loud and distorted.

Q: Distorted in what way?

A: Amplified sounds may seem unnatural, particularly if they are louder than you are accustomed to hearing them. Have you ever heard music so loud or distorted that you couldn't recognize the tune? The same thing can happen to sounds that are amplified by a hearing aid.

Q: How?

A: Since a hearing aid does not recognize specific sounds, it cannot selectively amplify sounds in a given frequency. You may need amplification in a certain frequency to understand whispered conversation but not to hear other, louder sounds in that frequency. But the hearing aid amplifies not only the whisper, but the other sounds as well. So while the whisper might sound just right, the water running from your kitchen faucet might sound like a tidal wave.

Q: Do you mean hearing aids amplify sounds that don't need to be amplified?

A: Hearing aids are designed to amplify all sounds in the frequencies to which they are tuned. Thanks to new technology, special features and options are available to reduce the problems this causes, but the amplification of background noise is still a problem for many hearing-aid wearers. Background noise suddenly becomes audible, and since many hearing-aid wearers have not been able to hear this noise for a long time, they must learn to tune out the noise all over again.

Q: It sounds like there are a lot of problems with hearing aids. Why should I even bother?

A: Because a hearing aid can vastly improve your hearing. Imagine being able to hear sounds you haven't recently been able to, listening to the radio at less than high volume or being able to participate in conversations. Hearing aids do make your hearing better. They simply cannot make it perfect. If you expect a hearing aid to restore your hearing, you will be disappointed.

Q: Is that why many people resist using hearing aids?

A: It is one reason, yes. The other reasons generally relate to cosmetic or psychological issues. There is a common belief that hearing aids are big and clunky and will detract from a person's physical appearance. And many people either don't want to believe that they have a hearing problem, or don't want others to know. It is estimated that only between 8 and 18 percent of those with hearing loss have a hearing aid, despite the fact that hearing aids could benefit a much higher percentage.

Q: Can hearing aids benefit everyone with hearing loss?

A: No. The benefits derived from hearing aids vary according to the severity and frequency of hearing loss, as well as the style of the hearing aid. Certain styles will not work for severe hearing loss, and hearing aids will not benefit people with loss in certain higher frequencies.

Q: In which frequencies are they useful?

A: Generally, hearing aids are useful in the lower frequencies. People with hearing problems in frequencies 1,000 Hz or lower will probably benefit from a hearing aid. And those whose loss occurs at frequencies near 1,500 Hz may be helped. But if the loss occurs at about 2,000 Hz or above, chances are a hearing aid will be of little use. Remember, most sounds made in conversation are below 2,000 Hz, so a loss in the 2,000 Hz range may not cause serious communication problems. Because you may not hear consonant sounds such as f, s, th, t and k, you may miss a word here and there, but you've probably learned to cope. A hearing aid might not be appropriate.

Q: What if you have hearing loss in both ears? Do you need two hearing aids or is one enough?

A: Experts generally recommend two hearing aids for people with bilateral hearing loss. Binaural hearing helps you localize sound, estimate your distance from the source of the sound, deal with more than one sound at a time and tune out background noise. Two hearing aids better prepare a wearer to hear sounds coming from both the right and the left and make sound seem more balanced.

Still, there are instances where a single hearing aid is more appropriate. If one ear has no measurable hearing at all, for example, or one "good" ear processes speech well, a single aid may be more appropriate. Consult with your doctor, audiologist or hearing-aid dealer to learn what is right for you.

Q: How do hearing aids work?

A: Different types of hearing aids work in different ways, but all hearing aids have three major components: a microphone, which picks up sounds; an amplifier, which makes them louder; and a speaker or receiver, which transmits the sounds to the ear. Basically, a hearing aid is a miniature sound system, powered by a tiny battery.

Hearing-Aid Types

Q: What are the different types of hearing aids?

A: Technological advances during the past few years have greatly expanded the selection of hearing aids. Not too long ago, the only type of hearing aid available was an **analog** hearing aid, which converts sound into an electronic signal. Now, there are three basic circuitry types available. In addition to analog circuitry, there is **digital** circuitry, which converts the electronic signals into numerically coded signals, like those used in computer microchips. There is also a **hybrid** circuitry, which combines analog and digital technology. In these devices, digital computer chips control the operation of the analog components.

Digital technology has also made it possible for hearing aids to actually be programmed like a computer. A small microchip, containing the programs needed to tailor the hearing aid to its user, can be placed inside the **digitally programmable** aid.

Q: **With all that technology, are there any advantages to an analog aid?**

A: An analog aid comes with a choice of special options and can be somewhat customized for its wearer. It has a long, successful track record and is generally less expensive than the other types.

Q: **What are the disadvantages?**

A: Analog aids do not usually offer the same number of special feature options offered by digital or programmable aids. Their sound clarity may not be as good, and they tend to make *all* sounds louder.

Q: **What about digital aids? What are their advantages?**

A: Digital aids provide better sound clarity and are generally more flexible than analog aids, because there are more special feature options available. They are designed to reduce background noise and provide better volume control and can be programmed to automatically adjust for loudness and reduce background noise.

Q: **And the disadvantages?**

A: For one thing, they are more expensive than analog aids. They are usually larger as well. And their effectiveness has received mixed reviews. Despite their elaborate technology and higher cost, digital aids have not shown significant benefit over the analog and hybrid aids. While some improvements have been reported in understanding speech if the speaker is talking in the higher frequencies and the background noise is in the lower frequencies, there is little improvement when the background noise contains a mixture of frequencies.

Q: **What advantages to do the hybrids have?**

A: They are as effective as the analogs, but they are more adaptable.

Q: Any disadvantages?

A: The hearing aid cannot be reprogrammed or adjusted to correspond with the wearer's changing needs without being sent back to the factory.

Q: How about the digitally programmable hearing aids? What are their advantages?

A: Digitally programmable hearing aids can be custom-tailored to your personal needs and listening environment. The hearing-aid dealer can program the aid to amplify different frequencies to different degrees. In addition, these devices may contain other programs stored in the memory of a microchip. Some aids, for example, can be programmed to adjust to up to eight different listening environments, such as a noisy restaurant or quiet car. The user simply pushes a button on the hearing aid or a remote control to call up the correct program. And when the user's needs change, the hearing-aid dealer can reprogram the aid right in his office.

Q: Sounds like an expensive product?

A: It is. Programmable aids are several times more expensive than analog aids. Many also rely on remote controls—which can be lost or broken—for adjustments and programming. Also, the devices use more power, so their batteries must be changed frequently.

HEARING-AID TYPES

Type	Description
Analog	Converts sound into electronic signals; special options available; reliable; may amplify all sounds; least expensive.
Digital	Converts electronic signals into numerically coded signals, like those used in computer microchips; more special options available; reduces background noise; better volume control; larger; more expensive.
Hybrid	Combines analog and digital technology —digital computer chips control the operation of analog components; reliable; adaptable; must be sent to factory for adjustment.
Digitally programmable	Uses digital technology and computer microchips to tailor the device to its user; can be custom-programmed; can be adjusted for different environments; may rely on remote control; most expensive.

Hearing-Aid Styles

Q: Did you say that hearing aids also come in different styles?

A: Yes, they do. There are five basic hearing-aid styles, varying in size and shape, and the location in which the aids are worn. Most of today's hearing aids are of three styles—behind-the-ear,

in-the-ear or in-the-canal. Eyeglass and body
hearing aids, the other two styles, are becoming
increasingly rare.

Q: Why? Don't they work?

A: Remember, vanity can play a very important
role in a person's decision whether or not to get
a hearing aid. It can also affect a person's choice
of style. The eyeglass and body hearing aids,
among the first styles available, work but are
considered either inconvenient or cosmetically
unacceptable by most people.

Q: What is unacceptable about eyeglass aids?

A: Eyeglass aids, designed to conceal the hearing
aid in the temple cover of the eyeglass frame,
require you to wear your glasses. The devices
make your glasses heavy and limit your choice
of frame. Further, the eyeglass aids are not an
option for contact lens wearers or people
without vision problems, and they are useless
when you remove your glasses.

Q: And body aids?

A: These very visible, powerful devices are worn
somewhere on the body, then connected to the

ear via wires and receivers. They are now used primarily for people with severe hearing impairment, particularly children.

Q: **What about the more common styles? Are any of them falling out of favor?**

A: Yes, the behind-the-ear style, standard in the 1960s and 1970s, is losing some of its popularity to the newer, smaller in-the-ear and in-the-canal styles. In fact, only about 15 percent of hearing-aid wearers now opt for the behind-the-ear style.

Q: **Is the behind-the-ear style too big and clunky or doesn't it work well?**

A: Behind-the-ear aids are durable, versatile and work very well, but they are somewhat obvious. No doubt you've seen many. These aids are arc-shaped and fit behind the ear. They are connected to the ear with a small piece of tubing that connects to the **earmold**, a piece of plastic that fits snugly in the ear.

Q: **What are the advantages of a behind-the-ear hearing aid?**

A: There are several. They are effective, durable and versatile. Their larger size provides space for a variety of special features to be built into the circuitry. A number of assistive listening devices, such as the **telecoil** circuit or T-switch, are designed to be used with them and their controls are easy to manipulate. They can be used for any degree of hearing loss, from mild to severe.

Q: **What are the disadvantages?**

A: The primary disadvantage, according to many people, is their size. While they have gotten considerably smaller in recent years, behind-the-ear aids are still more conspicuous than smaller types. They can also be uncomfortable for people who wear glasses or have ears that are close to the head. And because the microphone is positioned outside the ear, it can pick up and amplify wind and similar environmental sounds.

Q: **Are the newer styles that much better?**

A: Acoustically, no. But they are smaller and more readily accepted. The growth in the number of hearing-aid users has been attributed in part to the advent of the in-the-ear style.

Q: **What does the in-the-ear style look like?**

A: In-the-ear aids fit into the opening of your ear, right outside the ear canal. The parts are contained in a case that is custom-made to match the contours of your ear.

Q: **Is the in-the-ear style effective for all levels of hearing loss?**

A: Its smaller size makes it inadvisable for people with severe hearing loss, but those with mild, moderate or moderate-to-severe loss often benefit from an in-the-ear aid. Still, since the appropriateness varies with the degree and configuration of an individual's hearing loss, anyone considering an in-the-ear aid should consult with an audiologist or hearing-aid dealer to find out what his particular situation dictates.

Q: **What are the advantages of in-the-ear aids?**

A: The smaller size is the biggest advantage, in that many people find the size more cosmetically appealing. In addition, a number of special features can be added to customize the aid.

Q: **Are there any disadvantages?**

A: Ironically, the smaller size can work against the in-the-ear aid. Its amplification power is more limited than behind-the-ear aids, and its controls are smaller, which may make adjustment difficult for some people. Space for special features is rather limited. And because the microphone and receiver are close together, there can be a problem with **acoustic feedback**—squealing caused by amplified sound leaking out and being reamplified.

Q: Does the small size cause similar problems in in-the-canal aids?

A: Yes, it does. In fact, the amplification power of in-the-canal aids is only strong enough to compensate for mild to moderate hearing loss. The controls are difficult to adjust, room for special features is even more limited and acoustic feedback is often a problem. In-the-canal aids also require more cleaning and repairs because earwax builds up on the components.

Q: Are there any advantages to in-the-canal aids?

A: One: They are barely visible.

Q: Do they fit entirely in the ear canal?

A: Actually, they fit into the space at the beginning of the ear canal and extend slightly into the canal.

Q: Can you get an in-the-canal aid with digital circuitry?

A: Yes. In fact, all three of the common hearing-aid styles can be purchased with digital, analog or hybrid circuitry, so you can choose both your type and style.

HEARING-AID STYLES

Style	Description
Behind-the-ear	Arc-shaped device that fits behind the ear and connects to an earmold in the ear; appropriate for all degrees of hearing loss; room for many special feature options; durable; largest; least expensive.
In-the-ear	Round device, enclosed in custom-fitted case that fits in the opening of the ear outside the canal; appropriate for mild, moderate and moderate-to-severe hearing loss; limited amplification power; less space for special features; small controls; may produce acoustic feedback; small; mid-priced.
In-the-canal	Small round device, enclosed in case custom-fitted for the ear-canal opening; appropriate for mild to moderate hearing loss; limited amplification power; little space for special-feature options; small controls; may produce acoustic feedback; requires more repairs; smallest; most expensive.

Choosing a Hearing Aid

Q: **With all these choices available, how can I decide what type and style of hearing aid to get?**

A: Several factors should figure into your decision: the degree and frequencies of your hearing loss, your need for special features, your manual dexterity, your personal preference, and of course, the cost.

Q: **Now for the bad news. What can I expect to pay for a hearing aid?**

A: The cost of a hearing aid varies anywhere from about $500 to more than $2,000, depending on the circuitry type (analog, hybrid, digital or digitally programmable), style (behind-the-ear, in-the-ear or in-the-canal) and brand. The cost can double if you need a hearing aid for each ear.

Q: **Does the price include the special features that can be added to customize the hearing aid?**

A: No. The prices of the options, which we'll discuss later, run anywhere from $50 to $1,000.

Q: Why are hearing aids so expensive?

A: That's a good question. The actual cost of the components in a standard analog hearing aid is very low. Items such as a microphone, magnetic receiver, transistors, resistors, capacitators, wire and plastic are readily available and inexpensive. Microchips and other digital hearing-aid components obviously are more expensive. But you're not simply buying components. Labor, advertising and distribution add to the manufacturer's cost, and he sells the finished product to the retailer at a profit. The real markup, however, comes from the retailer.

Q: Why does the retailer charge so much?

A: The obvious answer is to make money. Selling at a profit is, of course, the role of a retailer. But there's more to it than that. When you buy a hearing aid from a hearing-aid dealer or dispenser, you are not simply buying an electronic device. You are also buying a package of services.

Q: What kind of services?

A: The dispenser is responsible for fitting you for the hearing aid, testing to make sure the hearing aid is correcting the problem, teaching you how to operate and care for the hearing aid and routinely servicing the aid. In some cases, the dispenser also does the initial hearing evaluation and provides an aural rehabilitation program to help you adjust to your hearing aid.

Q: **Are these services also provided for lower-priced models?**

A: In most cases, yes.

Q: **Well then, let's get back to the cost. What might a behind-the-ear aid cost?**

A: According to *Consumer Reports* (November 1992), you can purchase a decent behind-the-ear analog aid for between $500 and $700. This price includes a 30-day follow-up visit, a six-month checkup and a one-year warranty. A behind-the-ear aid with several options will cost between $700 and $1,000, and an aid with digital circuitry between $1,000 and $1,200. The higher-tech digitally programmable behind-the-ear aid will run anywhere from $1,200 to $2,000.

Q: **How about an in-the-ear aid?**

A: *Consumer Reports* says you may be able to purchase an in-the-ear aid for as little as $700. Most of the standard in-the-ear aids run between $700 and $1,000. For $1,000 to $1,200, you can get an analog aid with several options or a low-cost digital aid. A digitally program-mable in-the-ear aid will run $1,200 to $2,000.

Q: What would an in-the-canal hearing aid cost?

A: Prices for in-the-canal aids, which generally cost an average of $100 to $200 more than other styles, start at between $700 and $1,000, again according to *Consumer Reports*. Digitally programmable in-the-canal aids cost between $1,200 and $2,000.

Q: Whew! And some of those are without options! What do the more popular options cost?

A: Compared to the cost of the hearing aids them-selves, some of the options are reasonable. For about $50, for example, you can add a push–pull or power circuit, which can make a hearing aid helpful for persons with very severe hearing loss; a telecoil, which helps people talk on the phone without feedback; or compression, which keeps loud sounds from being overamplified.

Other options are more expensive. Automatic gain control, which helps control background-noise distortion and keeps loud sounds from becoming too loud, without requiring the wearer to adjust the volume, costs between $100 and $150, for example, while the popular

K-Amp, which amplifies soft and medium sounds without amplifying loud sounds, costs between $100 and $200. The most expensive option is a remote-control device for digitally programmable aids, which costs between $400 and $900. This control enables the user to switch the various programs off and on.

Q: **How many of these options do most people get?**

A: That depends on their needs and the style of hearing aid they choose. Remember, the smaller aids have limited space for these options. Some of the options are available only for certain types of hearing aids, and others are designed specifically for certain types of hearing loss. Someone with mild hearing loss, for example, would have no need for a push–pull circuit. For common problems, a variety of options are available, which enables a consumer to comparison shop for the best value.

Q: **While we're still talking money, will my insurance plan cover the cost of my hearing aid?**

A: Probably not. Most private policies do not cover hearing aids, although they usually do cover hearing evaluations. You need to check with your insurance representative to find out what is and what is not covered. Medicaid—but not Medicare—will cover some of the costs of a hearing aid, and the Veterans Administration will cover some costs for veterans. Some state rehabilitation and senior-citizen agencies offer financial assistance as do some local nonprofit service organizations, such as Lion's, Kiwanis and SERTOMA clubs. There is also an organization, HEAR NOW, which provides hearing aids to those who need financial assistance. For more information, see the section "Informational and Mutual-Aid Groups."

Q: **This might come directly out of my pocket. How can I find the best bargain?**

A: Comparison shop. Prices vary tremendously from dealer to dealer. And since the dealer also provides services, make sure you're dealing with someone who is qualified to help you.

Choosing a Hearing-Aid Dealer

Q: How can I find a qualified dealer?

A: Shop around. Perhaps the doctor or audiologist who examined you sells hearing aids. If not, he may be able to recommend either an audiologist who sells hearing aids or a nonprofessional hearing-aid dealer with experience and training. If you must find an audiologist on your own, make sure she's certified. Remember, if she is, her title will include the letters CCC-A. The American Speech-Language Hearing Association, which certifies audiologists, or the American Academy of Audiology, the audiologists' professional organization, may be able to help you locate a qualified audiologist in your area.

If you decide to go to a dealer, make sure he is licensed or registered by the state. Nearly every state regulates hearing-aid dealers in some way (Colorado and Massachusetts are the exceptions). Check with the state licensing board or department of health for licensing or registration information. And try to find a dealer who is certified by the National Board of Certification of Hearing Instrument Scientists. Certified dealers have the letters BC-HIS in their title. The International Hearing Society, which oversees the board, may be able to help you find a certified dealer in your area. Contact them at 20361 Middlebelt Road, Livonia, MI 48152 or call 800-521-5247. You can also check with the local Better Business Bureau and the state attorney general to see if any complaints have been filed against the dealer. This may sound like a lot of work, but it can help avoid future hassles. Some dealers have been known to engage in questionable practices and pass themselves off as audiologists or doctors.

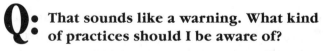

Q: That sounds like a warning. What kind of practices should I be aware of?

A: Over the years, a variety of hearing-aid scams have been perpetrated on people. Unscrupulous dealers have downplayed the need for hearing tests, convinced people without hearing problems that they need hearing aids and sold people hearing aids that do nothing for their type of hearing loss. They have engaged in misleading advertising, with the primary goal of getting into your house or convincing you to come to their office so they can do a hard sell. Free hearing tests and promises of free gifts have been used to lure people into this high-pressure, hard-sell trap.

Q: Did I hear that advertising is also a problem?

A: Yes. In fact the U.S. Food and Drug Administration in 1993 issued official warnings to six major hearing-aid manufacturers: Dahlberg, Inc., which makes the Miracle Ear line; Siemens Hearing Instruments; Omni Hearing Systems; Starkey Laboratories, Inc.; Beltone Electronics Corp.; and Electone, Inc. The FDA ordered them to stop making misleading claims in their advertisements.

Q: Like what?

A: The ads included unsupported claims that one product is markedly superior to another, that hearing aids can eliminate background noise and that hearing aids can restore hearing to its youthful quality.

Q: **Are there any regulations regarding the sale of hearing aids?**

A: Yes. Because of these problems, the FDA established regulations in 1977. The major provision prevents dealers from selling hearing aids to an individual unless she presents a signed statement from her physician indicating that she has had a hearing test within the past six months and that she may need a hearing aid.

Q: **Then how are dealers selling hearing aids to people who don't need them?**

A: Very easily. The regulations allow people over 18 to waive the medical evaluation. And while the dealer is required by law to advise the buyer not to waive the evaluation, many do not. In fact, many bury the required waiver statement somewhere in pages of paperwork, so that the buyer does not know what she is signing.

Q: **Are there any other sales practices I should be aware of?**

A: Yes. Purchasing hearing aids from door-to-door salespeople or through the mail presents its own unique problems. Determining the proper type of hearing aid and obtaining the proper fit are difficult in both situations, and the door-to-door salesperson may not be around later.

Q: Do I have any recourse if I order a hearing aid from a door-to-door salesperson or a mail-order company?

A: You have several rights as a consumer. The Federal Trade Commission's Door-to-Door-Sales Rule gives you the right to cancel any sale for $25 or more within three business days. And the Mail Order Rule requires companies to ship purchases when promised or give consumers the option to cancel their order and receive a refund.

Q: Do you have any other advice for selecting a dealer?

A: Yes:

• Try to avoid those that sell only one type or brand of hearing aid.

• Choose only from dealers who offer at least a 30-day trial period.

• Try to find a dealer who offers or can recommend an aural rehabilitation program—training to help you adjust to your new hearing aid.

• Before you buy anything, make sure you know what the price includes and what the warranty includes.

HOW TO AVOID HEARING-AID SCAMS

1. Have your ears examined and evaluated by a doctor or a certified audiologist before buying a hearing aid.

2. Avoid purchasing a hearing aid from a door-to-door salesperson.

3. Avoid purchasing a hearing aid through the mail.

4. Purchase your hearing aid from a certified audiologist or from a dealer that is licensed or registered by the state.

5. If you buy from a dealer, make sure he is certified by the National Board of Certification of Hearing Instrument Scientists.

6. Check with the local Better Business Bureau and state attorney general to find if any complaints have been filed against the dealer.

7. Be wary of the hard sell. Free hearing tests and promises of free gifts have been used to lure people into a high-pressure sales pitch.

8. Be wary of claims in hearing-aid advertisements. No hearing aid can totally eliminate background noise or restore hearing to its youthful quality.

9. Make sure your dealer offers a 30-day trial period.

10. Make sure you know exactly what hardware and services are included in the purchase price and what is covered by the warranty.

Buying a Hearing Aid

Q: What happens after I've found a reputable dealer?

A: That depends. If you've already had your hearing thoroughly evaluated, the dealer will examine your test results, discuss your options and help you try different hearing aids. If you have not had your hearing evaluated, the dealer will test your hearing. We've already discussed the different types of hearing tests. Remember, a hearing evaluation should include both pure-tone and speech-discrimination tests.

Q: What type of questions should I ask at this point?

A: You need to know what each particular hearing aid can and cannot do. Ask:

- about its sound quality;
- whether it will help in quiet places or noisy places;
- whether it is easy to operate;
- how it can be adjusted;
- what types of special features can be added to it;
- whether it is comfortable;
- what it costs to maintain;
- any other bit of information you feel will help you make your decision.

Q: What happens after I decide which type of hearing aid I should get?

A: You will be fitted. Remember, the earmold of a behind-the-ear hearing aid, as well as the casing of the in-the-ear and in-the-canal aids, is custom-fitted to the shape of your ear so that it will be comfortable and not cause acoustic feedback. The dealer makes an impression of your ear which is used to make the earmold or casing.

Q: So I probably won't get my hearing aid that day, will I?

A: Probably not. It may take a week or more to get your hearing aid. The earmold or casing must be custom-made, and some of the special feature options must be factory-installed.

Q: Okay, I've got my hearing aid. What now?

A: Your dispenser will help you put it in, make sure it fits and teach you how to operate it. You need to know how to insert and remove it, how to turn it off and on, how to adjust the volume, how to change the batteries and how to clean and care for it. The dispenser should be able to teach you these procedures.

Q: Am I on my own then?

A: Not quite. You still need to know how well the hearing aid is working. Your dispenser should perform a series of aided hearing tests on you—hearing tests in which you wear your hearing aid.

Q: What do these tests tell?

A: The tests determine how well you hear tones and speech with your aid and measure how loud the hearing aid makes sounds.

Q: Do these tests have specific names?

A: Yes. The first is called a **functional gain test**, and it is similar to the pure-tone tests you take prior to purchasing a hearing aid. The second is called a **real-ear measurement**. A miniature microphone is placed behind the hearing aid to measure its output to the eardrum.

Q: Are any other tests done?

A: Speech-discrimination tests may or may not be done.

After the Purchase

Q: Okay, the tests show my hearing aid is working fine. Will I have any other contact with my dealer?

A: If you have questions, concerns or problems; if your hearing changes and your hearing aid needs to be adjusted accordingly; or if your dealer schedules a future checkup, offers **aural rehabilitation** or services hearing aids, you will see him again.

Q: What is aural rehabilitation?

A: An aural rehabilitation program will help you adjust to your hearing aid. If you've grown accustomed to living with hearing loss, you may find life with a hearing aid very different. Background noises that you once took for granted suddenly seem like they are blaring from loudspeakers. It takes time to learn how to tune out unwanted sounds. An aural rehabilitation program will help you pick out speech against a variety of background noises. It will also teach you other methods for coping with hearing loss and offer counseling and support.

Q: What kind of servicing can dealers do?

A: Many dealers can clean, dry and replace parts of hearing aids, and most can also make minor tuning and programming adjustments when needed. Dealers who do not service hearing aids may send the aid to the manufacturer for servicing.

Q: All that talk about service! Aren't hearing aids reliable?

A: The reliability of a hearing aid depends both on the hearing aid itself and on how it is maintained. Hearing-aid quality varies greatly among brands. Higher quality aids can be very reliable, while low-quality devices can break repeatedly. Reliability can also vary with the style of the hearing aid. In general, the smaller hearing aids are less reliable than behind-the-ear aids. Because the smaller aids are situated in or near the ear canal, wax can build up on the components. This brings up the question of maintenance. A hearing aid's reliability is also dependent on its being kept clean and handled carefully.

Q: What kind of things can go wrong with a hearing aid?

A: Hearing aids can get clogged with wax, be dropped, get wet or get dirty, especially if used every day. Some of the components are fragile and tiny and can be affected by regular wear and tear.

Q: **Does the warranty cover repairs and servicing?**

A: It depends on the warranty. The FDA requires manufacturers to provide at least a one-year warranty on all new hearing aids, but there are no specific requirements about what the warranty must include. The terms of that warranty should be spelled out in the purchase agreement.

Q: **What do I use when my hearing aid has been sent back to the manufacturer for repairs?**

A: Many dealers will loan you a hearing aid during this time. Ask about a loaner before you purchase your hearing aid.

Q: **How long does a hearing aid last?**

A: Usually between three and five years.

Q: And then?

A: Then you buy another one. Or, if you know your hearing has changed, you have your hearing reevaluated and start all over again.

OTHER DEVICES

Cochlear Implants

Q: Are any other prosthetic devices available for the hearing impaired?

A: Yes. In recent years, a device has been developed that allows individuals with profound sensorineural hearing loss—actually, deafness—to "hear" certain sounds. This device is called a **cochlear implant**.

Q: What does this device do?

A: A cochlear implant is an electronic prosthesis that partially replaces some functions of the cochlea. Rather than amplifying sound like a hearing aid, it translates sounds into electrical impulses and delivers them straight to the auditory nerve.

Q: What does this device consist of?

A: A cochlear implant consists of one or more electrodes implanted in or adjacent to the cochlea, a stimulator/receiver which is also implanted, and a speech processor.

Q: But the cochlea is in the inner ear. Wouldn't this require surgery?

A: Yes, it would. The surgery is performed under general anesthesia and usually lasts two to three hours. The skin behind the ear is lifted; a mastoidectomy is performed; the middle ear is entered and the cochlea is opened so the electrode can be inserted. A processor is then coupled to the implant.

Q: This sounds like an expensive procedure. Is it?

A: Yes. Because this technology is relatively new, the cost of the implant alone ranges from $14,000 to $18,000. The surgery and rehabilitation cost an additional $6,000 to $10,000.

Q: Rehabilitation? What for?

A: A cochlear implant does not reproduce sounds the way we hear them. Only certain sounds, such as sirens, horns and doorbells, can be heard, although improvements to the processor have begun to make it possible to understand some speech with a cochlear implant. Still, interpreting these sounds, particularly after hearing nothing, requires rehabilitative training.

Q: **Can these devices really help people who are totally deaf?**

A: Yes, in fact they are used exclusively in people who are profoundly deaf in both ears—people who have an auditory threshold above 90 decibels.

Q: **Can they be used in children?**

A: The FDA approved the implants for use in adults in 1984 and in children in 1990, but cochlear implantation for children is controversial.

Q: **Why? Isn't the ability to hear linked to speech development?**

A: Yes. And ironically, that's the problem. While a cochlear implant would enable children to hear sound, theoretically enabling them to develop speaking skills, deaf children have no previous experience with sound and are difficult to rehabilitate. Cochlear implants are most effective in people who at one time had the ability to hear.

Assistive Listening Devices

Q: What devices are there, other than hearing aids, that can help the hearing impaired?

A: Many so-called assistive listening devices on the market make it easier to hear sounds in certain situations. They include: **infrared, FM** and **loop systems**, which transmit sound from a specific location directly to the ears; systems to improve telephone communications; **tele-captioning**, which allows hearing-impaired individuals to read the audio portion of a television program or video; and **assistive alerting devices** and **assistive signaling devices**, which alert hearing-impaired people to important sounds by either loud noises or visual signals.

Q: Wait a minute—one at a time! What exactly is an infrared system and where is it used?

A: An infrared system, used in theaters, concert halls, auditoriums and other large rooms, uses infrared light rays to transmit sound to receivers. These receivers can be hooked into headsets or hearing aids. Basically, it enables the sound to get to the people who need it before it dissipates.

Q: Are the FM and loop systems similar?

A: In terms of what they accomplish, yes. The FM system uses FM radio signals to transmit sound, while the loop uses a microphone and amplifier attached to electrical wire.

In the FM system, which is used primarily in classrooms and lecture halls, the speaker talks into a microphone, which is in fact a tiny radio transmitter. The sound is broadcast throughout the room and is picked up by receivers worn by the listeners.

In the loop system, which is also used in classrooms and lecture halls, an electrical wire is put in a circle around the area where the enhanced sound is needed. The electrical current creates a magnetic field that can be picked up by a hearing aid with telecoil circuitry—the T-switch.

Q: What kind of devices exist to enable the hearing impaired to better access telephones?

A: Several amplification devices are available, including an amplification wheel located on the volume control of the telephone's handset. This wheel can increase the telephone's volume by 30 percent. There is also a battery-operated portable amplifier. The T-switch, or telecoil circuit, one of the more common hearing-aid options, enables hearing-aid wearers to use the phone and their hearing aid simultaneously by making the hearing aid's circuitry compatible with that of other electronic devices. A new device, the videophone, can help hearing-impaired individuals who can read lips. And there is a Telecommunications Device for the Deaf **(TDD)**, which enables profoundly deaf people to communicate using the phone lines.

Q: How does the TDD work?

A: The device, hooked onto its own phone line, connects the line to a typewriter. Hearing-impaired individuals can dial a TDD number and converse via typewritten messages. It's similar to sending electronic mail from a computer over the phone lines to another computer.

Q: Is telecaptioning the same as closed captioning?

A: Yes. When you look in your television guide, you often see the letters CC after a program listing. This means the program is closed-captioned for the hearing impaired. Closed-captioned programs carry a written text of the dialogue on television programs. This dialogue runs under the picture, much like subtitles in a foreign film. Hearing-impaired people are able to read the dialogue and not miss any of the action.

Q: I've seen those listings, but the captions haven't appeared on my screen. Why not?

A: To receive the captions, you need a decoder or a television with built-in decoder circuitry. Since July 3, 1993, all new televisions with 13-inch or larger screens have been required to include the built-in circuitry.

Q: You mentioned assistive alerting and signaling devices. What are they?

A: Assistive alerting devices are loud bells, buzzers and ringers that enable hearing-impaired people to be alerted to important sounds like smoke or fire alarms, crying babies or medical emergencies. Assistive signaling devices also alert, but in a visual or other sensory manner. Flashing lights, vibrating devices and fans can all be hooked up to alert hearing-impaired individuals to important sounds.

Q: Aren't dogs able to do the same thing?

A: Yes, they are. Hearing-ear dogs can alert their owners to important sounds, either visually or through the sense of touch. But since these dogs also provide companionship and are not actually devices, we'll discuss them in the next chapter, when we discuss other methods of coping with hearing loss.

5 COPING WITH HEARING LOSS

Q: Does hearing loss affect anything other than hearing?

A: It certainly does. Hearing loss can affect speech and language development in infants and young children and has an obvious affect on communication later in life. As a result, it can affect a person's relationships with others. And its emotional and social effects can include isolation, loneliness and depression.

HEARING LOSS IN CHILDREN

Q: We touched on this before, but how does hearing loss affect speech and language development?

A: Children learn to speak based on what they hear. They imitate sounds and words, learning the meanings through experience. If they cannot hear or cannot hear well, they do not have the models they need. In short, they have nothing to imitate. This is why children with profound hearing loss have difficulty adjusting to cochlear implants. They have no previous experience with sound—nothing with which to compare the new sounds they are hearing. It is also why some deaf children never learn to speak.

Q: Can anything be done to help?

A: Early detection of hearing problems is crucial. If the problem can be corrected early, there may be little effect on speech and language development. Even if the loss is permanent, early detection and early intervention strategies can minimize the effect. Hearing aids, special education programs and work with a **speech-language pathologist** are all possible options.

Q: What is a speech-language pathologist?

A: A speech-language pathologist is an allied health professional who identifies specific problems in speech and provides nonmedical therapy to correct them. Speech-language pathologists measure and evaluate language abilities and speech production and treat people with language disorders. Often found in schools, hospitals and rehabilitation centers, they can help hearing-impaired children learn to speak correctly and help hearing-impaired adults retain their speaking skills. They can also work with deaf children to teach them the language and help them learn to speak.

Q: **What kind of methods do they use?**

A: Speech-language pathologists use a variety of methods that depend on the actual problems they are addressing. When working with a deaf child, for example, their goal may be to help the child become aware of the few sounds he may be able to hear, learn to recognize words, then sentences, and learn the meanings of those words. They may accomplish the first of these goals by repeating two different noises—say a bell and a whistle—until the child can differentiate between them and know which sound is produced by which object. Similar differentiation exercises may be done for words and sentences. To teach the meanings of words, they may perform actions while saying the words, or use a variety of other exercises.

For children who have difficulty making specific sounds, a speech-language pathologist may teach the child to recognize those sounds. Imitation and discrimination exercises may be used. The child may be asked to repeat what he has heard or recognize the difference between two words. Speech-language pathologists may also help the child form those sounds, explaining how they are made, manipulating the child's face, giving cues as to where the tongue should be or where the mouth should be positioned, while they are saying the words.

Q: Does it require a lot of training to be a speech-language pathologist?

A: Speech-language pathologists must have at least a master's degree in speech-language pathology. If they wish to be certified by the American Speech-Language Hearing Association (which also certifies audiologists), they must also complete 350 hours of supervised clinical experience and pass a written examination. A certified speech-language pathologist will have the letters CCC-SP after his name. This stands for Certificate of Clinical Competence in Speech-Language Pathology. Some individuals earn certification in both audiology and speech-language pathology. They can be identified by the CCC-SP/A title.

Q: Does hearing loss also affect a child's learning in areas other than speech and language?

A: It may. For deaf children, language deficiencies may make it difficult to learn other concepts. It's hard to understand a concept when it is explained in a language you don't understand. But even for children who know the language, hearing loss can have a detrimental effect on learning. In a traditional school setting, much of the material is presented verbally. Instructions, too, are usually given verbally. A student who can't hear well—one with chronic ear infections, for example—may miss large amounts of information and misunderstand instructions. Since few children have the confidence to continuously ask their teacher to repeat instructions, hearing-impaired students may fall behind. That's why it's important to be alert to the possibility that your child has a hearing problem.

Q: **You talked about how to tell if a young child has hearing loss; are there any signs to look for in an older child?**

A: Some of the signs are the same as those for younger children and adults: mispronouncing common words or speaking too loudly or too softly, for example. Children with hearing loss may also have frequent earaches, make mistakes when following verbal directions, frequently ask people to repeat themselves or appear to be inattentive. They may answer questions in irrelevant ways and imitate others rather than implement action themselves.

Q: **What should parents do if they suspect their child is hearing impaired?**

A: First and foremost, they should make sure their child is examined and tested. Hearing problems that can be corrected should be taken care of as soon as possible. If the problem cannot be corrected, the child's otolaryngologist or audiologist should be consulted to determine the best course to follow to help the child communicate and learn. They may be able to recommend speech-language pathologists, special education programs, counselors and support groups that can help both the child and the parents adapt to the situation. Once a plan of action has been determined, routine hearing evaluations can help monitor the progress of treatment or the progress of the loss, so that the plan can be adjusted accordingly.

Q: **What can parents do to help their child adapt to hearing loss?**

A: Parents of a hearing-impaired child need to be both supportive and patient. They need to understand the difficulties their child must face on a daily basis and work to minimize them. Making it easier for their child to communicate with them is an obvious first step. If the child is deaf, parents might learn **sign language**, **fingerspelling** or whatever method of communication the child uses. In any case, parents should learn and practice standard strategies for communicating with the hearing impaired. These strategies, which we'll discuss in detail shortly, include speaking in ways which will maximize the child's comprehension and improving the listening environment.

Parents can adapt their homes, adding carpets, drapes or wall hangings to improve the **acoustics** or investing in assistive listening devices, such as telephone amplifiers or signaling devices. They should also inform school officials and teachers about their child's problem and work with them to find ways to make learning easier for their child.

Q: Are there any specific things that can be done to help a hearing-impaired child in the classroom?

A: Yes. Once a teacher is aware of the problem, she can make things easier for the child in a number of ways. She can seat the child in the front of the class, away from fans, hallways, windows and other sources of external noise, to make it easier for the child to hear what is being said. She can face the child when she is talking, so that he can watch her facial expression and mouth. She can also supplement the material she presents verbally with written worksheets or study sheets, write assignments on the board, and try to improve the acoustics of the classroom.

Q: What about deaf children? How are they taught?

A: Deaf children can either be taught at schools for the deaf or in regular schools. At schools for the deaf, specially trained teachers work with the students. In regular schools, the students can either attend special classes led by specially trained teachers; or standard classes, where they are helped by tutors, resource teachers and, if they communicate with sign language, interpreters. The actual methods for teaching deaf students depend on the communication methods the students use. If they use sign language, for example, the teacher can instruct in sign language. If they speech read, the teacher can practice standard communication strategies and supplement instruction with written material.

Q: **I assume that children with hearing problems might have emotional and social problems to overcome as well, right?**

A: Right. Because they probably miss so much of what's going on around them, they may feel isolated. Because they may not be able to participate in conversation, their friends may feel ignored, and ignore them in return. Because they misunderstand what is said and respond incorrectly, their teachers and peers may think they lack intelligence. And the children, in turn, may become self-conscious and lack self-confidence. Of course, hearing-impaired adults can face similar problems.

Q: **But adults at least understand what's happening to them, don't they?**

A: They should, but often they don't. Hearing loss in adults often comes on gradually. It may not become noticeable until it reaches the moderate or severe level, and even then it may be noticed only by the individual's friends and family.

Q: Why?

A: For one thing, it's hard to know you haven't heard something if you haven't heard it. For another, people who gradually lose their hearing develop and become dependent on coping mechanisms without even realizing it. Finally, many individuals simply refuse to admit they have a problem. They deny that they can't hear and instead blame others. They may ask, for example, why everyone is whispering, or accuse others of mumbling.

Q: Why would they do that?

A: They may look at their hearing loss as a sign of weakness or vulnerability and not want to "need help," or they may be afraid of how it will change their lifestyle. After all, it is difficult for most people to accept shortcomings or handicaps they have not had to cope with in the past.

Q: Don't denying the problem and transferring the blame cause social problems?

A: They can. When well-meaning friends or family members recognize a problem and suggest that help should be sought, they do not expect their concern to be dismissed or repaid with accusations. Even when they understand the psychological reasons behind those reactions, they can put strain on a relationship.

COMMUNICATION

Q: Do other factors affect a hearing-impaired individual's relationships with others?

A: Yes. Communication is the cornerstone of most relationships, and since hearing loss has a profound affect on communication, relationships are often affected.

If you're talking to a hearing-impaired person, it can be irritating to be asked to repeat yourself continuously or to be misunderstood. It takes more time to converse. Friendly conversation becomes a chore. You get frustrated. And you might not even know why you're having this difficulty. You might think your friend simply isn't listening or doesn't care. Eventually, you may stop communicating with him altogether.

If you are the one who is hearing impaired, conversation is not simply a chore, it's hard work. You must give it your undivided attention. You often must strain to hear and understand. Even then you may have to ask for clarification. You get tired, perhaps embarrassed. You sense your friend's impatience and frustration. You become frustrated yourself. Eventually, you may simply try to communicate less. You may withdraw.

Q: That can lead to loneliness, right?

A: Right. Many hearing-impaired individuals, embarrassed or frustrated by their inability to communicate, simply stop socializing. They withdraw from their circle of friends, turn down invitations or participate only minimally. And they end up feeling lonely, isolated and, often, depressed.

Q: **Are there ways to make communication easier so that these social and emotional problems can be avoided?**

A: There certainly are. A number of coping mechanisms exist, which, like hearing aids and assistive listening devices, can make communication, and life in general, easier for the hearing impaired. The listening environment can be improved. Friends and family can be taught strategies that make their speech easier for a hearing-impaired individual to understand, and hearing-impaired individuals can learn to speech read or use sign language.

Strategies for Friends and Family

Q: **What can I do make it easier for a hearing-impaired individual to understand me?**

A: First, remember that missing sounds and distracting background noises are the roots of the problem, not inattention or lack of interest. In fact, most hearing-impaired people probably pay more attention than people with normal hearing—they have to to get by. Don't get upset if your friend misunderstands or asks you to repeat yourself. Instead, take the problem by the roots—work with your friend to fill in the sound gaps and improve the listening environment.

IMPROVING THE LISTENING ENVIRONMENT

Q: What can I do to improve the listening environment?

A: First of all, be conscious of it. Background noises that you might be able to "tune out" could make it difficult for your friend to "tune in" to your conversation. The primary goal is to reduce these noises so that your friend can concentrate on the conversation.

Q: What can I do to reduce background noise in my home?

A: Make sure your rooms are carpeted and your windows covered by drapes. Both carpeting and drapes absorb sound and improve a room's acoustics. Choose appliances and toys that are quiet. Whenever possible, place fans, air conditioners and other noisy appliances in out-of-the-way places. Turn off the television, radio and other nonessential appliances before you begin a conversation, and never speak to your friend from another room.

While we're talking about the house, you should also make sure that the rooms in which you converse are well lit. This will not minimize background noise, but it will make it easier for your friend to see who's talking.

Q: What can I do outside of my home?

A: Basically, you want to duplicate your home's listening environment as much as possible. Choose rooms with carpeting and drapes; find areas to converse that are away from fans, televisions and other noisy appliances and stay away from large, noisy groups.

If you're going out to eat, for example, choose a quiet restaurant—one without televisions blaring or a loud band—and request a table away from the kitchen, where clattering dishes and employees' conversations may be distracting. Ask for a corner table, and have your friend sit in the corner. The acoustics are better there. If no corner table is available, choose a table near the wall, away from large groups of people. In theaters, churches or lecture halls, sit where your friend can take advantage of any available assistive listening devices. If there are no devices, sit near the front, close to the source of sound. And no matter where you are, when you talk to your friend, make sure he can see your face.

Q: What sort of devices are you talking about?

A: Primarily the loop, infrared and FM systems we discussed in the last chapter. Depending on which system is used, your friend should sit either in the loop or near a receiver.

SPEAKING STRATEGIES

Q: What can I do to help my friend understand what I'm saying?

A: First and foremost, make sure he knows you are speaking to him.

- Get his attention.

- Face him when you speak.

- Speak clearly and slowly.

- Make sure he understands what you've said before you move on.

- Use gestures and facial expressions, but don't cover your mouth while you speak.

- Don't talk while you're eating or chewing gum.

- Don't change the subject abruptly.

- Ask if there are any other things you can do to help him understand you.

Q: A lot of people raise their voices when talking to hearing-impaired people. Should I?

A: If you've been whispering, yes. But in general, no. Whatever you do, don't shout. When you shout, the hearing-impaired individual might hear you, but chances are what you've said will sound distorted to him. It's like shouting in English at someone who speaks a foreign language. It won't help him understand, and it will make both of you feel uncomfortable.

Q: **Should I just keep repeating until he understands?**

A: Let's take the foreign language metaphor one step further. No matter how many times you repeat a phrase, if the listener doesn't know the meaning of the words you're repeating, it will make no sense to him. The same thing applies to a hearing-impaired individual. If he cannot figure out which words you're repeating, he cannot understand what you're saying. Your best bet is to try to rephrase what you want to say. Perhaps other words are easier for him to hear.

Strategies for the Hearing Impaired

Q: **I'm hearing impaired. What strategies can I use to improve communication?**

A: It is difficult for anyone without an impairment to fully understand the problems of a person with hearing loss. First, you must let others know you have a hearing problem. Make them aware of your specific needs, so that they can adapt to them. In a sense, you must act as an educator. You may also want to improve your

listening and communication abilities and your
listening environment.

Q: **Do I need to make strangers aware of my
hearing problem?**

A: Strangers won't be aware of your problem or
know how to adapt to your needs unless you tell
them. If you want to improve your communication with them, you have to inform and
educate them. While time-consuming, this can
make your life easier. In emergencies, it may do
more than that—it may make your life possible.

Q: **Why? Aren't emergency personnel familiar
with hearing impairment?**

A: While many hospitals and doctors' offices have
educated their employees about communicating
with the hearing impaired, others have not.
And even if medical personnel are aware of
communication strategies, they may not be
aware of your particular problems or methods
of communicating.

Q: **What exactly do they need to know?**

A: They need to know that you are hearing impaired and to what extent. They also need to

know how you deal with your impairment and how you communicate. They need to know, for example, if you wear a hearing aid, if you rely on speech reading or if you communicate with sign language.

Q: **But I may be one of many patients. How will they remember all those details?**

A: Many hospitals and doctors' offices have established specific methods to deal with hearing-impaired patients. They mark the patient's chart, records, identification bracelet or nameplate with a sticker, so that all of the medical professionals who have dealings with him are aware of the situation and can adapt their communication methods accordingly.

Q: **What should I do if I'm in a hospital or doctor's office that hasn't established a program?**

A: Be assertive. Post your own hearing-impaired sign and remind employees that they must adapt to communicate with you. Remind them how important it is for patients—all patients—to understand explanations and instructions. And above all, don't be afraid to ask for clarification when you need it. Understanding can mean the difference between life and death.

Q: What are some other instances when it's helpful to educate others about my hearing impairment?

A: It's a good idea to "turn teacher" whenever you want to avoid costly communication mistakes. If you're traveling, for example, and don't understand the flight announcements, you could miss your plane. Letting someone know about your problem and working with that person to obtain the information you need could save you both time and money. Don't be shy. Ask the flight attendant if you've boarded the correct plane so you don't head in the wrong direction; ask a stranger to write down the directions he's just given you so you can avoid hours of backtracking and panic; and ask a salesclerk for clarification and written terms in a complicated purchase so you can prevent a future trip to the return counter.

IMPROVING THE LISTENING ENVIRONMENT

Q: How can I improve my listening environment?

A: The primary goal is to keep background noise to a minimum so that it is easier to concentrate on conversation. This is accomplished in different ways in different environments. We touched on these methods when we listed strategies for family and friends, but since they also apply to the hearing impaired, they bear repeating here.

Q: Let's start at home. How can I minimize background noise in my house?

A: Make sure your rooms are carpeted and your windows covered by drapes. Both carpeting and drapes absorb sound. Cloth wall hangings, too, may improve your home's acoustics. Choose appliances and toys that are quiet. Whenever possible, place fans, air conditioners and other noisy appliances in out-of-the-way places.

While we're talking about adapting the house, you should also make sure that the rooms in which you wish to converse are well lit. This won't minimize background noise, but it will make it easier to see who's talking.

Q: What if I'm away from home?

A: When you're not at home, look for areas that duplicate your home's listening environment as much as possible. Choose rooms with carpeting and drapes; find areas to converse that are away from fans, televisions and other noisy appliances; stay away from large, noisy groups and other sources of noise, and get as close as possible to the source of the sounds you are trying to hear.

In theaters, churches and lecture halls, for example, sit where you can take advantage of the assistive listening system or, if there is no system, near the front. When you go out to eat, choose a quiet restaurant—one without televisions blaring or a loud band—and request a table away from the kitchen, where clattering dishes and employees' conversations may be distracting. Ask for a corner table and sit in the corner. The acoustics are better there.

Q: **Where else can I position myself so that I can hear better?**

A: Corners are the best; near a wall is also good. Whenever possible, stay away from noise and large groups. Stand near the people you want to talk to, and position yourself so that you can see their faces. Talk only with people who are in the same room with you; never shout from room to room.

LISTENING AND COMMUNICATION STRATEGIES

Q: **What else can I do to help others communicate better with me?**

A: Remember, you're the teacher. Don't be afraid to ask others to speak slowly, speak louder, repeat what they've said or do anything else that will help you understand them. You might also learn to speech read.

Speech Reading

Q: What is speech reading?

A: Speech reading is using visual clues to understand what is being said. A hearing-impaired individual watches the lips and face of a speaker to help determine what was said.

Q: Isn't that the same as lip reading?

A: Yes and no. In the past, speech reading was called lip reading. But speech readers look at much more than lips. Facial expressions and gestures also play a key role. Even for people with normal hearing, it is estimated that up to 40 percent of speech comprehension is visual. This is one reason that it may take hearing-impaired people time to recognize their problem. They may be depending on these visual clues to get by without even noticing that their hearing is deteriorating.

Q: How does speech reading work?

A: The hearing-impaired individual positions herself so that she can see who is speaking. She keeps her eyes on the speaker's face when he speaks, watches his lips to see what words he is forming, and listens for key words and phrases to determine the context. She also watches the speaker's facial expressions and gestures and listens for inflections and other nuances that may provide clues to what is being said. A rising inflection at the end of a sentence might indicate a question, for example, while a loud word might be stressed for emphasis.

Q: That sounds like a lot of work! What kind of results does it get?

A: Speech reading is a lot of work, but many people find that it is worth the effort. Still, speech reading is not foolproof. A number of words and sounds may look alike. The sounds b, p and m, for example, are all formed with lip movements that look identical to a speech reader. Thus, the words ban, pan and man would all look identical. This is when context becomes important. Context is also important when the speaker uses sounds such as n, d, t, g, k and ng, which are made without any visible lip movement.

A backup technique called **cued speech** can also be used to overcome these problems. In cued speech, while speaking, the speaker makes a manual sign that clarifies sounds the speech-reader cannot distinguish. Of course, this requires the speaker to learn the cues.

Q: Is it difficult to learn to speech read?

A: Not really. In fact, you probably already know how to speech read to some extent. To see just how much you depend on your eyes for comprehension, try this simple test. Sit down with a friend in a noisy setting and talk for a while. Look at him while you're talking. Then ask him to hold something in front of his face. Chances are he will be much more difficult to understand when you can't see his face.

Q: So can I just learn speech reading naturally?

A: You can. In fact, many people teach themselves, learning from experience. But formal instruction is also available. There are books that outline techniques and provide practice exercises. And there are classes that teach techniques and help you fine-tune your skills. To find a class, check with your otolaryngologist, audiologist or speech-language pathologist, or check the communication disorder center or speech pathology department of a university or hospital near you. The Alexander Graham Bell Association for the Deaf, Inc., 3417 Volta Place N.W., Washington, DC 20007, 202-337-5220, may also be able to help you locate a speech-reading class in your area.

Q: **Can people with hearing aids benefit from speech reading?**

A: Many times, yes. Remember, a hearing aid does not restore perfect hearing. There may still be gaps in conversation. Speech reading can help fill in those gaps.

Q: **How about the deaf? Can they speech read?**

A: Some can and some cannot. It depends to a large extent on their familiarity with the English language. If they lost their hearing early, before their language abilities were fully developed, chances are they will have difficulty with speech reading. If they lost their hearing later in life, after years of using the language, they may find speech reading very helpful.

Q: **Are there any other ways I can improve my communication ability?**

A: Ask people to spell words you cannot understand when spoken. Communicate in writing. And, if your hearing loss is profound, consider learning sign language.

Manual Communication

Q: Tell me more about sign language. What exactly is it?

A: Sign language—or, to be more exact, sign languages—is a form of **manual communication**. Used primarily by the deaf and those who wish to communicate with them, sign language involves making gestures and signs with the hands that are seen visually, so that language can be seen rather than heard. These strategies, which have been used for thousands of years, have been adapted into a number of different systems or languages and are used throughout the world.

Q: How many different forms of sign language are used in the United States?

A: There are at least six in common use—**American Sign Language** and a number of systems that can be described as **manually coded English**, or **manual English**.

Q: What do you mean by manual English?

A: Manual English systems take the English language and literally translate it into manual gestures. Manual English systems use both signs and fingerspelling; the signs and gestures correspond to English words and a manual alphabet is used to spell out English words. And the language structure—word order and syntax—parallels that of English.

Q: **What are the names of these manual English systems?**

A: The most common manual English systems are: Signed English, Seeing Essential English (SEE I), Signing Exact English (SEE II), Linguistics of Visual English (LOVE) and Pidgin Signed English (PSE). Pidgin Signed English also uses some characteristics of American Sign Language.

Q: **How does American Sign Language differ from manual English?**

A: American Sign Language (ASL), the language of the deaf, is not based on English. It is its own language with its own grammar and syntax.

Q: **Is ASL difficult to learn?**

A: That depends on a person's language-learning ability. Learning ASL is similar to learning any other foreign language. It takes time, practice and effort to become fluent.

Q: **Doesn't that deter people from learning it?**

A: It certainly does. While ASL is picked up as a first, or primary, language by most of the people who are born deaf or who lose their hearing at an early age (between 100,000 and 500,000 Americans consider it their primary language), people who lose their hearing later in life rarely learn it. Like the majority of hearing people who need to communicate with the deaf or hearing impaired, if they decide to learn a sign language, they choose a manual-English system rather than ASL.

Q: **Are there any other factors that deter people from learning ASL?**

A: Yes. Up until the 1960s, when ASL was determined to be an actual language, its use was discouraged and, in some cases, forbidden. Educators were concerned that it would interfere with the learning and use of English, because its grammar and structure are different. Now that it is viewed as a language of its own, and ASL users have shown that they can also learn English, some of the resistance has subsided. But the acceptance of ASL has generated a cultural controversy that deters some people from it.

Q: What's the controversy?

A: There is a debate among the deaf community about ASL. Some view it as a unique language that gives identity to the deaf culture, while others believe it secludes and isolates them, since few hearing people use it. This debate mirrors the debate over sign language itself.

Q: What is that debate?

A: The debate centers around whether or not the deaf should adapt their communication strategies to correspond with those of the hearing world. Some people believe that the deaf must be taught to speak and speech read; others believe they should be taught to communicate manually, through sign language. Sign-language supporters maintain that sign language provides an adequate communication system for the deaf. They don't believe the deaf should be forced to adapt to the standards of the hearing world.

Supporters of the "oral approach," on the other hand, argue that sign language, while enabling the deaf to communicate, can actually isolate them, since it is not widely used in the hearing world. They believe it is better for the deaf to learn and use English so they can function in the hearing world.

Q: Isn't there any compromise?

A: While the debate rages, some people have attempted a compromise. One approach has the deaf speak and sign simultaneously. And popularity is also growing for another approach, called **total communication**. In total communication, deaf people are encouraged to communicate using any and every method available to them. This means they can sign, speech read, use hearing aids and other amplifying devices, speak, fingerspell, draw or write.

Q: I guess it's a matter of individual choice, isn't it?

A: It is. There are several choices to be made, all of which can affect your future communication strategy. You need to weigh the pros and cons of sign language, in general, and determine if it's right for you. If it is, you must decide which language to learn. Finally, you need to spend the time and effort to learn the language and practice it until you become fluent.

Q: Where can I learn sign language?

A: Sign language classes are available nearly everywhere. Community colleges, colleges, universities, churches, local park and recreation offices, rehabilitation centers and speech and hearing centers often offer classes. Check your newspaper for announcements, check the course lists of local colleges, or pick up a phone book and start dialing. Call the community colleges, look under the language-communication services listing of the human services section or check the yellow pages under "Rehabilitation Services." You could also check with your audiologist, speech-language pathologist or a representative of a local support or self-help group to see if he knows where classes are held.

OTHER COPING MECHANISMS

Q: **Switching the subject, what about hearing-ear dogs. Do they really help the hearing impaired cope?**

A: Hearing-ear dogs do indeed provide a valuable service that can help their owners cope with daily life and regain or retain their independence: They alert their owners to important sounds which might otherwise go undetected.

Q: **How do they alert their owners?**

A: The dogs make physical contact with their owners to alert or signal them to specific sounds. Most dogs can alert their owners to up to six sounds, according to the Service Dog Center, which provides information about hearing-ear and other service dogs. The most common are: a doorbell, a knock at the door, a telephone ring, a smoke alarm, a baby crying, an alarm clock and the person's own name. But dogs can also be taught to respond to other sounds, such as a dryer or microwave beep.

The dogs usually are trained to touch their owners, then lead them to the source of the sound. In the case of the smoke alarm, they are taught to alert their owners in a different manner, so that the owners immediately know they are dealing with a possible emergency.

Q: **Where are these dogs trained?**

A: Training, which takes from four months to a year, can be done at a training center, by a private trainer or by a hearing-impaired dog owner. Center training is handled in several ways, according to the Service Dog Center. In some cases, the dog is trained at the center, then its owner visits the center for a period of time to learn to work with the dog; in other cases, the trainer and trained dog come to the new owner, and in still other instances, the dog and its owner go through training together. A private trainer can work with the dog and its owner at home or at the trainer's place of business. And more and more people are training their own dogs, which can be faster, since the demand for hearing-ear dogs exceeds the supply.

Q: What breeds make the best hearing-ear dogs?

A: Any breed, even a mixed breed, will do as long as the dog is intelligent, eager to please, has high energy and can localize sound. Most of the dogs trained by centers tend to be small to medium-size, according to the Service Dog Center. But larger dogs have also been trained and can make good hearing-ear dogs.

Q: Where do these dogs come from?

A: That depends. Some centers specifically breed dogs to train; others train dogs rescued from animal shelters, and personal pets trained by their owners come from a variety of sources.

Q: What can you expect to pay if you get a hearing-ear dog from a center?

A: The cost of a hearing-ear dog varies. Some centers charge nothing; some charge a good-faith fee and some charge the cost of training the dog, which can be up to $5,000. But financial assistance is usually available.

Q: How can I find a training center?

A: The Service Dog Center, P.O. Box 1080, Renton, WA 98057-9906, 206-226-7357, will give you names of centers in your area. If you're looking for more comprehensive information, the Center sells a service dog directory for $3, which includes the names and locations of training centers, the kinds of dogs they train and the kinds of services they offer.

Q: While we're on the subject of coping with daily life, how can a person cope with hearing loss on the job?

A: Good question. When hearing loss strikes before the retirement years, it can greatly affect a person's ability to do his job. Obviously, hearing aids, speech reading and other coping mechanisms may help. And depending on the work situation, other assistive listening devices in the workplace might help. Talk with your employer to see if the listening environment can be improved.

You can also consult the vocational rehabilitation agency in your state. This agency works to help people with disabilities keep their present jobs or retrain for new ones. You may be eligible to receive medical, hearing and vocational evaluations, as well as guidance, counseling, training services or financial assistance to purchase a hearing aid or assistive listening device or cover the cost of education

and retraining. The agency may also be able to
help you find a new job. You can contact the
agency by looking under "Rehabilitation" or
"Vocational Rehabilitation" in the state government listings of your phone book's yellow or
blue pages.

Q: **Where else might I find counseling
and support?**

A: Depending on where you live, there may be a
number of organizations in your community
that can help you deal with hearing loss and its
effects. Check your yellow pages for listings of
local counseling centers, churches, hospitals,
speech and hearing centers, rehabilitation
centers, special education programs and self-
help groups, such as a local chapter of Self-
Help for Hard-of-Hearing People (SHHH), which
has a national office at 7910 Woodmont Ave.,
Suite 1200, Bethesda, MD 20814, 301-657-2248.
A number of other national organizations also
provide information and support. For a list of
those organizations, see the section "Informational and Mutual-Aid Groups."

INFORMATIONAL AND MUTUAL-AID GROUPS

Alexander Graham Bell Association for the Deaf, Inc.
3417 Volta Place N.W.
Washington, DC 20007
202-337-5220

Provides information on hearing loss, oral communication and the availability of speech-reading lessons; promotes better understanding of hearing loss by the public.

American Academy of Audiology
1735 N. Lynn St., Suite 950
Arlington, VA 22209
703-524-1923
800-222-2336

Professional organization for audiologists. Provides information on hearing impairment and referrals to qualified audiologists.

**American Academy of Otolaryngology–
Head and Neck Surgery, Inc.**
One Prince Street
Alexandria, VA 22314
703-836-4444

Professional organization for otolaryngologists. Provides information about otolaryngology, pamphlets about medical problems of the ear and referrals to physicians.

American Society for Deaf Children
814 Thayer Ave.
Silver Spring, MD 20910
800-942-ASDC (voice/TDD)

Provides referrals for parents of deaf children and resource materials on deafness.

American Speech-Language-Hearing Association
10801 Rockville Pike
Rockville, MD 20852
301-097-5700
800-638-8255 ASHA helpline

Professional organization for audiologists and speech-language pathologists. Provides information on speech, language and hearing problems and referrals to qualified audiologists and speech-language pathologists.

Better Hearing Institute
5021-B Backlick Road
Annandale, VA 22003
703-642-0580
800-EAR-WELL

Provides educational brochures and pamphlets about hearing loss, hearing aids and hearing health-care providers.

Cochlear Implant Club International
P.O. Box 464
Buffalo, NY 14223
716-838-4662 (voice/TDD)

Provides information on cochlear implants to medical professionals and those who have or are considering cochlear implantation; offers fellowship and support through local support groups; publishes a quarterly magazine.

Deafness Research Foundation
9 E. 38th Street, 7th Floor
New York, NY 10016
800-535-3323
212-684-6556 (voice/TTY)

Provides information on hearing loss.

Dial-A-Hearing Screening Test
800-222-EARS

Provides a local telephone number for a free hearing screening over the phone.

The EAR Foundation
2000 Church Street
Box 111
Nashville, TN 37236
615-329-7809
800-545-HEAR

Offers educational programs and support services on hearing and balance problems; administers the Ménière's Network, a national network of patient support groups.

Hearing Education and Awareness for Rockers (H.E.A.R.)
P.O. Box 460847
San Francisco, CA 94146
415-773-9590

Offers information on hearing loss, tinnitus, hearing protection and hearing testing.

HEAR NOW
9745 E. Hampden Ave., Room 300
Denver, CO 80231-4923
303-695-7797
800-648-HEAR

Raises funds to provide hearing aids, cochlear implants and other equipment for financially needy hearing-impaired people and operates a national hearing-aid bank.

House Ear Institute
2100 W. Third St.
Los Angeles, CA 90057
213-483-4431

Conducts research and provides information relating to hearing loss and deafness.

International Hearing Society
20361 Middlebelt Road
Livonia, MI 48152
313-478-2610
800-521-5247 (Hearing-Aid Helpline)

Professional organization for hearing-aid dispensers; provides information on hearing aids and referrals to local hearing-aid specialists.

National Association of the Deaf
814 Thayer Avenue
Silver Spring, MD 20910-4500
301-587-1788 (voice)
301-587-1789 (TTY)

Provides information and services for the deaf and hearing impaired including: books, magazines, scholarships, youth programs and leadership programs; certifies teachers of American Sign Language; and sponsors a legal defense fund.

National Captioning Institute
5203 Leesburg Pike
Falls Church, VA 22041
800-533-9673
800-321-8337 (TDD)

Distributes TeleCaption Decoders; provides list of where decoders can be purchased and repaired.

National Information Center on Deafness
Gallaudet University
800 Florida Avenue N.E.
Washington, DC 20002
202-651-5051 (voice)
202-651-5053 (TDD)

Provides information about hearing loss and services available to the deaf and hearing impaired.

National Information Center on Hearing Loss
P.O. Box 1880
Media, PA 19063
800-622-EARS

Provides information on hearing health, referrals to otolaryngologists, audiologists and hearing-aid specialists.

NIDCD Clearinghouse
1 Communications Avenue
Bethesda, MD 20892-3456
800-241-1044 (voice)
800-241-1055 (TDD)

Clearinghouse for the National Institute on Deafness and Other Communication Disorders; offers publications about hearing loss, deafness and communication disorders; can provide information about specific topics relating to hearing loss, deafness and communication disorders via a computer database.

Self-Help for Hard-of-Hearing People (SHHH)
7910 Woodmont Avenue, Suite 1200
Bethesda, MD 20814
301-657-2248

Provides information, education, referral, advice and support to hearing-impaired individuals. Publishes bimonthly journal.

Service Dog Center
P.O. Box 1080
Renton, WA 98057
206-226-7357

Provides information about hearing-ear dogs.

TRIPOD
2901 N. Keystone Street
Burbank, CA 91504
818-972-2080 (voice/TDD)
800-352-8888 (voice/TDD) hotline
800-2-TRIPOD in California (voice/TDD)

Provides services to families with children with hearing loss and information on issues of concern to deaf and hearing-impaired people through its toll-free hotline, the Grapevine.

GLOSSARY

Acoustic feedback: Squeal produced by a hearing aid when amplified sound escapes and is reamplified.

Acoustic nerve: The auditory nerve.

Acoustic neuroma: A benign tumor of the acoustic nerve that grows in the ear canal.

Acoustic otoscope: A medical instrument used for examining the ear that reflects sound waves off the eardrum.

Acoustics: The qualities of a room that determine its ability to reflect sound waves.

Acoustic trauma: Loss of hearing caused by exposure to loud noise over a long period of time, an explosion, blow to the head or another accident.

American Sign Language: A form of sign language with its own grammar, vocabulary and syntax, used primarily by deaf Americans.

Analog: Type of hearing-aid circuitry which converts sound into electronic signals.

Assistive alerting device: A device which alerts a hearing-impaired individual to sound through a louder sound, such as a bell, whistle or horn.

Assistive listening device: Any device which helps a hearing-impaired individual hear; this includes devices which alert, signal, amplify or direct sound or represent sound visually.

Assistive signaling device: A device which alerts a hearing-impaired individual to sound through vision, touch or other senses.

Audiogram: A graph, made by an audiometer, which shows the frequency and decibel level at which a person begins to hear.

Audiologist: A professional trained in the identification, evaluation and nonmedical rehabilitation of hearing loss.

Audiometer: An electronic instrument used to test hearing and measure the conduction of sound through bone and air.

Auditory nerve: The eighth cranial nerve; it transmits information from the cochlea to the brain.

Aural rehabilitation: Training and rehabilitation to teach a hearing-impaired individual to cope with limited hearing or adjust to a hearing aid.

Auricle: The external part of the ear; the pinna.

Barotrauma: Injury to the ear caused by a sudden change in air pressure.

Basilar membrane: The membrane in the cochlea, where the hair cells are located.

Bilateral: Two-sided; referring to both ears.

Brain stem audiometry: Computerized test which measures the response of the brain stem to sound.

Cerumen: Earwax.

Cholesteatoma: An abnormal growth of skin, or cyst, in the middle ear. It occurs as a congenital defect or as a complication of otitis media.

Cilia: Hair cells in the cochlea.

Cochlea: The spiral-shaped part of the inner ear; it receives sound waves from the middle ear and transmits the information to the auditory nerve.

Cochlear implant: A device, which, when implanted into the cochlea, enables people with profound hearing loss to hear certain noises.

Conductive hearing loss: Type of hearing loss caused by something impeding the conduction of sound through the outer and/or middle ear.

Cued speech: A technique in which manual signs are used to back up speech reading.

Curette: A long, thin instrument with a hook at the end; used by doctors to clean earwax from the outer ear canal.

Decibel: A relative measurement of sound intensity or pressure; literally one-tenth of a bel; an increase of one bel is approximately double the loudness of a sound.

Digital: Hearing-aid circuitry in which sound is converted into numerically coded signals like those used in computer microchips.

Digitally programmable: A type of hearing aid with digital circuitry that can be programmed like a computer to tailor it to its user's needs.

Ear canal: The opening by which sound enters the ear.

Eardrum: Tympanic membrane; a flat membrane which separates the outer ear canal from the middle ear.

Earmold: A device that fits in the ear to connect a behind-the-ear hearing aid to the ear.

Earmuffs: Noise protection devices that cover the ears.

Earplugs: Noise protection devices that fit in the ear canal.

Electrocochleography: A computerized test that provides information about the functioning of the inner ear.

ENT: An ear-nose-throat specialist; otolaryngologist.

Eustachian tube: Tube which connects the ear to the nose-throat cavity; it equalizes pressure in the middle ear.

Exostosis: An abnormal growth on the surface of a bone in the ear; also known as surfer's ear.

Fingerspelling: A form of manual communication in which words are spelled out with the hands by means of symbols that represent the letters of the alphabet.

FM system: An assistive listening system in a room, in which sound is transmitted via FM radio waves to a receiver worn by the hearing-impaired individual.

Frequency: The number of vibrations a sound makes per second, measured in cycles per second, or Hertz; sounds with higher frequencies will have higher pitches.

Functional gain test: Pure-tone test used to determine hearing abilities when a hearing aid is worn.

Hertz: International unit for frequency; equal to one cycle per second.

Hybrid: A type of hearing-aid circuitry in which digital computer chips control the operation of analog components.

Incus: The anvil; the central of the three small bones in the middle ear.

Infrared system: An assistive listening system for a room in which infrared light rays transmit sound to receivers worn by hearing-impaired individuals.

Inner ear: That portion of the ear which contains the cochlea and the labyrinth.

Labyrinth: The part of the inner ear, consisting of fluid-filled semicircular canals, which controls balance.

Labyrinthectomy: Surgery in which the inner ear is removed.

Loop system: An assistive device for a room, in which a microphone and amplifier are attached to an electrical wire which circles the room and creates a magnetic field; hearing-impaired individuals wearing hearing aids with telecoil circuitry can pick up the magnetized sound.

Malleus: The hammer; the first of three small bones in the middle ear.

Manual communication: Any form of communication in which the hands, rather than the spoken word, are used to communicate; i.e., sign language and fingerspelling.

Manual English: A form of manual communication in which hand signs are used to represent English words; the grammar and syntax of English are also used.

Manually coded English: Manual English.

Mastoid: A portion of the temporal bone; found behind the ear.

Mastoidectomy: Surgical removal of all or part of the mastoid process.

Mastoiditis: An inflammation or infection of the mastoid bone or its air cells—spaces lined by mucous membrane in the mastoid bone.

Ménière's disease: An inner-ear disorder of unknown cause that results in periods of vertigo or dizziness, hearing loss, buzzing or ringing in the ear and nausea.

Middle ear: That portion of the ear that begins at the eardrum and includes the three ossicles.

Mixed hearing loss: Hearing loss that is both conductive and sensorineural.

Myringoplasty: Surgical repair of a ruptured eardrum with a tissue graft.

Myringotomy: Surgical procedure in which a small incision is made in the eardrum to relieve pressure or allow fluid to drain from the middle ear.

Ossicles: Three small bones in the middle ear that form a bridge connecting the eardrum with the oval window.

Otitis externa: An inflammation or infection of the outer ear or outer ear canal; swimmer's ear.

Otitis media: An inflammation or infection of the middle ear.

Otitis media with effusion: An inflammation or infection of the middle ear, in which fluid is present in the middle ear.

Otolaryngologist: A medical doctor who specializes in disorders of the head and neck, especially those relating to the ear, nose and throat.

Otologist: An otolaryngologist who subspecializes in disorders of the ear.

Otorhinolaryngologist: Old term for otolaryngologist.

Otosclerosis: A congenital condition in which abnormal bone growth forms in the inner ear; it can cause tinnitus and deafness.

Otoscope: An instrument used to examine the external ear canal, eardrum and ossicles; it consists of a light and a magnifying lens.

Ototoxic: A substance that has a bad effect on the auditory nerve or inner ear; a substance that is poisonous to the ear.

Outer ear: That portion of the ear that begins with the pinna and includes the ear canal.

Oval window: Opening in the inner wall of the middle ear through which sound is passed into the inner ear.

Permanent threshold shift: A change in the hair cells that permanently changes a person's hearing sensitivity.

Pinna: Auricle; the external part of the ear.

Presbycusis: Sensorineural hearing loss, usually gradual, caused by aging.

Profound: A hearing loss of 90 decibels or more.

Prosthesis: A device which replaces a missing part of the body or makes a part of the body work better.

Pure-tone audiometry: Hearing tests, using an audiometer, which measure a person's ability to hear pure tones.

Pure-tone threshold: The point at which a person is able to hear pure tones from an audiometer.

Real ear measurement: Test which measures a hearing-aid's output to the eardrum.

Rinne test: Tuning-fork test which determines whether hearing loss is sensorineural or conductive.

Sensorineural hearing loss: The type of hearing loss caused by damage to the inner ear or auditory nerve.

Sign language: A form of manual communication in which gestures and signs, in a specific pattern, are used to communicate.

Speech-discrimination tests: Oral-aural tests which determine what speech sounds a person can discriminate; the listener must repeat words and sounds spoken to him.

Speech-language pathologist: An allied health professional who measures and evaluates language and speech production abilities and clinically treats individuals with speech and language disorders.

Speech reading: A technique in which a hearing-impaired person watches a speaker's lips, face and gestures to determine what that person has said.

Stapedectomy: Removal and replacement of the stapes or a portion of the stapes; used to treat otosclerosis.

Stapes: The innermost of the three small bones in the middle ear.

Swimmer's ear: Otitis externa; an inflammation or infection of the outer ear.

TDD: Telecommunications Device for the Deaf; an assistive device with which the deaf can communicate over the telephone; typewritten messages are sent and received over the phone lines.

Telecaptioning: A system which allows the deaf and hearing impaired to understand the spoken portion of audiovisual programs; dialogue appears in written form below the picture.

Telecoil: A circuitry option that can be added to a hearing aid; the telecoil makes the hearing aid circuitry compatible with external electronic devices like the telephone.

Temporal bone: The large bone on either side of the head; includes the mastoid bone.

Temporary threshold shift: A temporary change in the hair cells as a response to noise that temporarily changes a person's hearing sensitivity.

Tinnitus: A ringing or buzzing in the ear.

Total communication: An approach to communication for the deaf in which the deaf individual is encouraged to use any form of communication available to him, including sign language, speech, hearing aids, assistive listening devices and speech reading.

Tympanic membrane: The eardrum; a flat membrane that separates the outer ear canal from the middle ear and carries sound vibrations to the bones of the middle ear.

Tympanometer: Machine which tests the function of the eardrum and middle ear.

Tympanoplasty: Surgical operation on the eardrum or ossicles to restore or improve hearing; used to repair a broken eardrum.

Tympanostomy: Surgical implantation of tubes in the eardrum used to prevent a buildup of air pressure and fluid in the middle ear and, thus, prevent recurrent middle-ear infections.

Unilateral: One-sided; in one ear.

Vertigo: Dizziness.

Weber's test: Tuning-fork test which determines which ear functions better.

SUGGESTED READING

Carmen, Richard. *Our Endangered Hearing: Understanding and Coping With Hearing Loss.* Emmaus, Pa.: Rodale Press, 1977.

Carmen, Richard. *Positive Solutions to Hearing Loss.* Englewood Cliffs, N.J.: Prentice-Hall, 1983.

Freese, Arthur S. *You and Your Hearing: How to Protect It, Preserve It and Restore It.* New York: Charles Scribner's Sons, 1979.

Grundfast, Kenneth, and Cynthia J. Carner. *Ear Infections in Your Child.* Hollywood, Fla.: Compact Books, 1987.

Himber, Charlotte. *How to Survive Hearing Loss.* Washington, D.C.: Gallaudet University Press, 1989.

Huning, Debbie, M.A., C.C.C.-A. *Living Well With Hearing Loss: A Guide for the Hearing-Impaired and Their Families.* New York: John Wiley & Sons, 1992.

Marty, David R. *The Ear Book: A Parent's Guide to Common Ear Disorders of Children.* Jefferson City, Mo.: Lang E.N.T. Publishing, 1987.

Prescod, Stephen V. *Audiological Handbook of Hearing Disorders.* New York: Litton Educational Publishing Co., Inc., 1978.

Rezen, Susan V., and Carl Hausman. *Coping With Hearing Loss: A Guide for Adults and Their Families.* New York: Dembner Books, 1985.

Schmidt, Michael A. *Childhood Ear Infections: What Every Parent and Doctor Should Know About Prevention, Home Care and Alternative Treatment.* Berkeley, Calif.: North Atlantic Books, 1990.

Shimon, Debra, A. *Coping With Hearing Loss and Hearing Aids.* San Diego, Calif.: Singular Publishing Group, Inc., 1992.

Suss, Elaine. *When the Hearing Gets Hard: Winning the Battle Against Hearing Impairment.* New York: Plenum Press, 1993.

Tannenhaus, Norra. *What You Can Do About Hearing Loss.* New York: Dell Publishing, 1993.

Thomsett, Kay, and Eve Nickerson. *Missing Words: The Family Handbook on Adult Hearing Loss.* Washington, D.C.: Gallaudet University Press, 1993.

Vernick, David M., M.D., and Constance Grzelka. *The Hearing Loss Handbook.* Yonkers, N.Y.: Consumers Union of the U.S., Inc., 1993.

APPENDIX A:

FIVE-MINUTE HEARING TEST

	Almost always	Half the time	Occasionally	Never
1. I have a problem hearing over the telephone.				
2. I have trouble following the conversation when two or more people are talking at the same time.				
3. People complain that I turn the TV volume too high.				
4. I have to strain to understand conversations.				
5. I miss hearing some common sounds like the phone or doorbell ringing.				
6. I have trouble hearing conversations in a noisy background such as a party.				
7. I get confused about where sounds come from.				
8. I misunderstand some words in a sentence and need to ask people to repeat themselves.				
9. I especially have trouble understanding the speech of women and children.				
10. I have worked in noisy environments (assembly lines, jackhammers, jet engines, etc.).				

(continued on the following page)

FIVE-MINUTE HEARING TEST
(continued from the previous page)

	Almost always	Half the time	Occasionally	Never
11. Many people I talk to seem to mumble or don't speak clearly.				
12. People get annoyed because I misunderstand what they say.				
13. I misunderstand what others are saying and make inappropriate responses.				
14. I avoid social activities because I cannot hear well and fear I'll reply improperly.				
15. *To be answered by a family member or friend:* Do you think this person has a hearing loss?				

SCORING

To calculate your score, give yourself three points for every time you checked the "Almost always" column; two for every "Half the time," one for every "Occasionally" and zero for every "Never." If you have a blood relative who has a hearing loss, add another three points. Then total your points.

The American Academy of Otolaryngology–Head and Neck Surgery recommends the following:
- 0 to 5 —Your hearing is fine.
      No action is required.
- 6 to 9 —Suggest you see an ear-nose-and-throat specialist.
- 10 and above —Strongly recommend you see an ear physician.

Reprinted with permission from the American Academy of Otolaryngology–Head and Neck Surgery, Inc., Alexandria, VA 22314

APPENDIX B:

IS MY BABY'S HEARING NORMAL?

More than 3 million American children have a hearing loss. An estimated 1.3 million of these are under three years of age. You, the parents and grandparents, are usually the first to discover hearing loss in your babies, because you spend the most time with them. If, at any time, you suspect your baby has a hearing loss, discuss it with your doctor.

Your baby's hearing can be professionally tested at any age. Computerized hearing tests make it possible to screen newborns. Some babies are in a higher risk category for having hearing loss than others. If you check any items on this list, your child should have a hearing test as soon as possible.

All children should have their hearing tested before they start school. This could reveal mild hearing losses that the parent or child cannot detect. Loss of hearing in one ear may also be determined in this way. Such a loss, although not obvious, may affect speech and language.

Hearing loss can even result from earwax or fluid in the ears. Many children with this type of temporary hearing loss can have their hearing restored through medical treatment or minor surgery.

In contrast to temporary hearing loss, some children have nerve deafness, which is permanent. Most of these children have some usable hearing. Few are totally deaf. Early diagnosis, early fitting of hearing aids and an early start on special educational programs can help maximize the child's existing hearing.

Use this simple list to answer the question "Is My Baby's Hearing Normal?"

DETERMINING IF YOUR CHILD HAS A HEARING LOSS

If you think that your child has a hearing loss, you might be right. The following checklist will assist in determining whether or not your child might have a hearing loss. Please read each item carefully and check *only* those factors that apply to you, your family or your child.

Risk Criteria—Check Each Item That Applies:

DURING PREGNANCY

____ Mother had German measles, a viral infection or flu.

____ Mother drank alcoholic beverages.

MY NEWBORN (Birth to 28 days of age)

____ Weighed less than 3.5 pounds at birth.

____ Has an unusual appearance of the face or ears.

____ Was jaundiced (yellow skin) at birth and almost had or did have an exchange blood transfusion.

____ Was in neonatal intensive care unit (NICU) for more than two days.

____ Received an antibiotic medication given through a needle in a vein.

____ Had meningitis.

MY FAMILY

____ Has one or more individuals with permanent or progressive hearing loss that was present or developed early in life.

MY INFANT (29 days to age 2 years)

____ Received an antibiotic medication given through a needle in a vein.

____ Had meningitis.

____ Has a neurological disorder.

____ Had a serious injury with a fracture of the skull with or without bleeding from the ear.

Response to the Environment (Speech and Language Development)

MY NEWBORN (Birth to 6 months)

____ Does not startle, move, cry or react in any way to unexpected loud noises.

____ Does not awaken to loud noises.

____ Does not freely imitate sound.

____ Cannot be soothed by voice alone.

____ Does not turn his/her head in the direction of my voice.

MY YOUNG INFANT (6 through 12 months)

____ Does not point to familiar persons or objects when asked.

____ Does not babble or babbling has stopped.

____ By 12 months is not understanding simple phrases such as "wave bye-bye" and "clap hands" by listening alone.

MY INFANT (13 months through 2 years)

____ Does not accurately turn in the direction of a soft voice on the first call.

____ Is not alert to environmental sounds.

____ Does not respond on first call.

____ Does not respond to sound or does not locate where sound is coming from.

____ Does not begin to imitate and use simple words for familiar people and things around the home.

____ Does not sound like or use speech like other children of similar age.

____ Does not listen to TV at a normal volume.

____ Does not show consistent growth in the understanding and the use of words to communicate.

WHAT YOU SHOULD DO

If you have checked one or more of these factors, your child may be *at risk* for hearing loss. *At risk* simply means there is a better than average chance of a hearing loss.

If your child is at risk, you should take him for an ear examination and a hearing test. This can be done *at any age,* as early as just after birth.

If you did not check any of these factors but you suspect that your child is not hearing normally, even if your child's doctor is not concerned, have your child's hearing tested by an audiologist and when appropriate, his speech evaluated by a speech and language pathologist. If no hearing loss exists, the test will not have hurt him. However, if your child does have a hearing loss, delayed diagnosis could affect speech and language development.

This checklist is not a substitute for an ear examination or a hearing test. Hearing loss can exist in children even though none of these checklist items are present.

Reprinted with permission of the American Academy of Otolaryngology–Head and Neck Surgery, Inc., Alexandria, VA 22314

INDEX

A

Acoustic feedback, defined,
91, 157
Acoustic nerve, defined, 15, 157
Acoustic neuroma
defined, 43, 157
treatment, 44
Acoustic trauma
defined, 46-47, 157
sensorineural hearing loss and,
46-47
Acoustics
defined, 157
parents' coping strategies,
122-23
Advertising, hearing-aid, 100
Aerobics, high-impact, hearing loss
and, 46
Age
hearing and, 17
hearing loss and, 12, 55
Ménière's disease and, 45
presbycusis and, 55-56
Air pressure. *See also* Barotrauma
hearing and, 17, 22, 38
pneumatic otoscope and, 60

Alcohol, Ménière's disease and, 45
Allergies
barotrauma and, 38
conductive hearing loss and, 24
otitis media and, 28, 30
Alport's syndrome, sensorineural
hearing loss and, 42
American Academy of
Otolaryngology–Head and
Neck Surgery, tympanostomy
and, 34-35
American Sign Language (ASL)
controversies, 143-45
defined, 157
generally, 141
learning, 142-43, 145-46
vs. manual English, 142
Amikacin, side effects, 47
Amoxicillin, otitis media and, 31-32
Analog hearing aids
costs of, 93-96
generally/defined, 82, 86, 157
pros/cons, 83
styles of, 92
Antibiotics
immunity to, 32